Infectious Diseases in Pregnancy

Editor

GEETA K. SWAMY

OBSTETRICS AND GYNECOLOGY CLINICS OF NORTH AMERICA

www.obgyn.theclinics.com

Consulting Editor
WILLIAM F. RAYBURN

December 2014 • Volume 41 • Number 4

ELSEVIER

1600 John F. Kennedy Boulevard • Suite 1800 • Philadelphia, Pennsylvania, 19103-2899

http://www.theclinics.com

OBSTETRICS AND GYNECOLOGY CLINICS OF NORTH AMERICA Volume 41, Number 4
December 2014 ISSN 0889-8545, ISBN-13: 978-0-323-32664-3

Editor: Kerry Holland
Developmental Editor: Stephanie Carter

Obstetrics and Gynecology Clinics (ISSN 0889-8545) is published quarterly by Elsevier Inc., 360 Park Avenue South, New York, NY 10010-1710. Months of issue are March, June, September, and December. Periodicals postage paid at New York, NY, and additional mailing offices. Subscription price per year is $310.00 (US individuals), $545.00 (US institutions), $155.00 (US students), $370.00 (Canadian individuals), $688.00 (Canadian institutions), $225.00 (Canadian students), $450.00 (foreign individuals), $688.00 (foreign institutions), and $225.00 (foreign students). To receive student/resident rate, orders must be accompanied by name of affiliated institution, date of term, and the signature of program/residency coordinator on institution letterhead. Orders will be billed at individual rate until proof of status is received. Foreign air speed delivery is included in all *Clinics* subscription prices. All prices are subject to change without notice. POSTMASTER: Send address changes to *Obstetrics and Gynecology Clinics*, Elsevier Health Sciences Division, Subscription Customer Service, 3251 Riverport Lane, Maryland Heights, MO 63043. **Customer Service: Telephone: 1-800-654-2452 (U.S. and Canada); 314-447-8871 (outside U.S. and Canada). Fax: 314-447-8029. E-mail: journalscustomerservice-usa@elsevier.com (for print support); journalsonlinesupport-usa@elsevier.com (for online support).**

Reprints. For copies of 100 or more of articles in this publication, please contact the Commercial Reprints Department, Elsevier Inc., 360 Park Avenue South, New York, New York 10010-1710. Tel.: 212-633-3874; Fax: 212-633-3820; E-mail: reprints@elsevier.com.

Obstetrics and Gynecology Clinics of North America is also published in Spanish by McGraw-Hill Interamericana Editores S.A., P.O. Box 5-237, 06500, Mexico; in Portuguese by Reichmann and Affonso Editores, Rio de Janeiro, Brazil; and in Greek by Paschalidis Medical Publications, Athens, Greece.

Obstetrics and Gynecology Clinics of North America is covered in *MEDLINE/PubMed (Index Medicus), Excerpta Medica, Current Concepts/Clinical Medicine, Science Citation Index, BIOSIS, CINAHL, and ISI/BIOMED.*

Printed in the United States of America.

Contributors

CONSULTING EDITOR

WILLIAM F. RAYBURN, MD, MBA
Distinguished Professor and Emeritus Chair, Obstetrics and Gynecology Associate Dean, Continuing Medical Education and Professional Development, University of New Mexico School of Medicine, Albuquerque, New Mexico

EDITOR

GEETA K. SWAMY, MD
Associate Professor, Division of Maternal-Fetal Medicine, Department of Obstetrics & Gynecology, Duke University, Durham, North Carolina

AUTHORS

HOMA K. AHMADZIA, MD, MPH
Fellow, Division of Maternal Fetal Medicine, Department of Obstetrics & Gynecology, Duke University Medical Center, Durham, North Carolina

BRENNA ANDERSON, MD, MSc
Associate Professor, Department of Obstetrics & Gynecology, Women & Infants Hospital, Alpert Medical School of Brown University, Providence, Rhode Island

RICHARD H. BEIGI, MD, MSc
Associate Professor of Reproductive Sciences, Divisions of Obstetric Specialties and Reproductive Infectious Diseases and Immunology, Department of Obstetrics, Gynecology, Reproductive Sciences, Magee-Womens Hospital of the University of Pittsburgh School of Medicine and Medical Center, Pittsburgh, Pennsylvania

IRINA BURD, MD, PhD
Associate Professor, Department of Gynecology and Obstetrics, Johns Hopkins Medical Institutions; Integrated Research Center for Fetal Medicine, Johns Hopkins Medical Institutions; Department of Neurology, Johns Hopkins Medical Institutions, Baltimore, Maryland

JILL K. DAVIES, MD
Associate Professor, Department of Obstetrics & Gynecology, Denver Health Medical Center, University of Colorado Denver School of Medicine, Denver, Colorado

MEGHAN DONNELLY, MD
Assistant Professor, Department of Obstetrics and Gynecology, University of Colorado Health, University of Colorado Denver School of Medicine, Aurora, Colorado

JAMES M. EDWARDS, MD
Department of Obstetrics & Gynecology, Duke University Medical Center, Durham, North Carolina

AZADEH FARZIN, MD
Assistant Professor, Department of Pediatrics, Integrated Research Center for Fetal Medicine, Johns Hopkins Medical Institutions; Assistant Professor, Department of Pediatrics, Johns Hopkins Medical Institutions; International Center for Maternal & Newborn Health, Johns Hopkins University, Baltimore, Maryland

JOSEPH L. FITZWATER, MD
Fellow, Division of Maternal-Fetal Medicine, Department of Obstetrics and Gynecology, University of Alabama at Birmingham, Birmingham, Alabama

REBECCA GARCIA-PUTNAM, MD
Department of Obstetrics & Gynecology, Duke University, Durham, North Carolina

CAROLYN GARDELLA, MD, MPH
Associate Professor, Division of Women's Health, Department of Obstetrics and Gynecology, University of Washington; Director of Gynecology, VA Puget Sound Medical Center, Seattle, Washington

R. PHILLIPS HEINE, MD
Associate Professor, Director, Division of Maternal Fetal Medicine, Department of Obstetrics & Gynecology, Duke University Medical Center, Durham, North Carolina

CLARK T. JOHNSON, MD, MPH
Instructor, Department of Gynecology and Obstetrics, Johns Hopkins Medical Institutions; Integrated Research Center for Fetal Medicine, Johns Hopkins Medical Institutions, Baltimore, Maryland

JULIE JOHNSON, MD
Clinical Assistant Professor, Department of Obstetrics & Gynecology, Women & Infants Hospital, Alpert Medical School of Brown University, Providence, Rhode Island

AMY P. MURTHA, MD
Department of Obstetrics & Gynecology; Division of Maternal Fetal Medicine; Department of Pediatrics, Duke University Medical Center, Durham, North Carolina

MARTHA W.F. RAC, MD
Department of Obstetrics and Gynecology, University of Texas Southwestern Medical Center, Dallas, Texas

JEANNE S. SHEFFIELD, MD
Department of Obstetrics and Gynecology, University of Texas Southwestern Medical Center, Dallas, Texas

ALYSSA STEPHENSON-FAMY, MD
Assistant Professor, Division of Maternal Fetal Medicine, Department of Obstetrics and Gynecology, University of Washington, Seattle, Washington

GEETA K. SWAMY, MD
Associate Professor, Division of Maternal-Fetal Medicine, Department of Obstetrics & Gynecology, Duke University School of Medicine, Duke University, Durham, North Carolina

ALAN T.N. TITA, MD, PhD
Professor, Division of Maternal-Fetal Medicine, Department of Obstetrics and Gynecology, University of Alabama at Birmingham, Birmingham, Alabama

Contents

> Pregnant women are at risk for the same infectious diseases as nonpregnant individuals and often have increased morbidity and mortality associated with infection. Thus, immunizing women during pregnancy with recommended vaccines provides direct maternal benefit. Furthermore, maternal immunization has the potential for both fetal and infant benefit by preventing adverse pregnancy outcomes and infection during early life through passive immunity. This article reviews current knowledge on the importance and benefits of maternal immunization, which are 3-fold: protecting the mother from antepartum infection; reducing poor pregnancy and fetal outcomes; and providing immunity for infants during the first few months of life.

> Influenza infections are an important global source of morbidity and mortality. Pregnant and postpartum women are at increased risk for serious disease, related complications, and death from influenza infection. This increased risk is thought to be mostly caused by the altered physiologic and immunologic specifics of pregnancy. The morbidity of influenza infection during pregnancy is compounded by the potential for adverse obstetric, fetal, and neonatal outcomes. Importantly, influenza vaccination to prevent or minimize the severity of influenza infection during pregnancy (and the neonatal period) is recommended for all women who are or will be pregnant during influenza season.

> Contemporary management of HIV in pregnancy remains a moving target. With the development of newer antiretroviral agents with lower side-effect profiles and laboratory methods for detection and monitoring of HIV, considerable progress has been made. This review examines key concepts in the pathophysiology of HIV and pregnancy with emphasis on perinatal transmission and reviews appropriate screening and diagnostic testing for HIV during pregnancy. Current recommendations for medical, pharmacologic, and obstetric management of women newly diagnosed with HIV during pregnancy and for those women with preexisting infection

Of the 5 types of viral hepatitis (HAV–HEV), HBV and HCV are by far the most common causes of chronic hepatitis in both pregnant and nonpregnant populations, causing more than 50% of cirrhosis cases and 78% of cases of primary liver cancer. Infection during pregnancy can have adverse effects on both the mother and her fetus. For all 5 viral hepatitis syndromes, early identification allows appropriate measures to be taken to optimize pregnancy outcomes and minimize the risk of perinatal transmission. This article reviews the prevention and management of all 5 viral hepatitis syndromes during pregnancy.

Congenital cytomegalovirus (CMV) is a leading cause of permanent disability in children. The main source of maternal infection is from contact with young children. Primary maternal infection is diagnosed with demonstration of seroconversion or a positive CMV IgM in combination with a low-avidity CMV IgG. Fetal infection may be diagnosed with amniotic fluid polymerase chain reaction and culture. CMV-specific hyperimmune globulin has shown promise as a possible means to prevent congenital infection; large randomized trials are ongoing. To date, the only effective means of prevention is through reducing exposure to the virus. Rates of maternal infection may be reduced through education regarding sources of infection and improved hygiene.

Genital herpes in pregnancy continues to cause significant maternal morbidity, with an increasing number of infections being due to oral-labial transmission of herpes simplex virus (HSV)-1. Near delivery, primary infections with HSV-1 or HSV-2 carry the highest risk of neonatal herpes infection, which is a rare but potentially devastating disease for otherwise healthy newborns. Prevention efforts have been limited by lack of an effective intervention for preventing primary infections and the unclear role of routine serologic testing.

Genital mycoplasmas are frequently found in the vaginal flora across socioeconomic and ethnic groups and have been demonstrated to be involved in adverse perinatal outcomes. Both *Mycoplasma* and *Ureaplasma spp* cause inflammation potentially leading to spontaneous preterm birth and PPROM as well as postdelivery infectious complications and neonatal infections. Herein we have provided an overview of the existing literature and supportive evidence for genital mycoplasma's role in perinatal complications. Future research will need to focus on clearly delineating the species, allowing for discrimination of their effects.

Group B streptococcus (GBS) can cause significant maternal and neonatal morbidity. Over the past 30 years, reductions in early-onset GBS neonatal sepsis in the United States have been attributable to the guidelines from the Centers for Disease Control and Prevention for antepartum screening and treating this organism during labor. This article highlights the clinical implications, screening, diagnosis, prophylactic interventions, and future therapies for mothers with GBS during the peripartum period.

Chorioamnionitis is the process of active infection within the amniotic cavity that induces an inflammatory response. A wide variety of pathologic organisms can cause chorioamnionitis. Prompt diagnosis and timely treatment with broad-spectrum antibiotics can help avert the significant short-term and long-term consequences that may result. This review aims to summarize the up-to-date diagnosis criteria, treatment protocols, and long-term sequelae of missed diagnoses or poorly treated disease. It also calls for future studies that aim to better understand the mechanism of disease and to develop better detection and intervention methods to prevent the significant associated morbidity.

Cesarean wound infections represent a significant health and economic burden. Several modifiable risk factors have been identified for their development. Understanding these risks and techniques to manage cesarean wounds is essential for providers. In this article, these factors and prophylactic and therapeutic interventions are reviewed.

OBSTETRICS AND GYNECOLOGY CLINICS

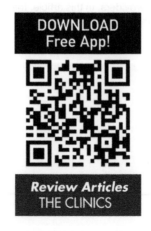

DOWNLOAD
Free App!

Review Articles
THE CLINICS

NOW AVAILABLE FOR YOUR iPhone and iPad

Foreword

Infectious Diseases in Pregnancy

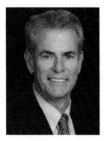

William F. Rayburn, MD, MBA
Consulting Editor

Infectious disease is the single most common medical condition encountered by the obstetrician. This issue of *Obstetrics and Gynecology Clinics of North America*, edited by Dr Geeta Swamy, updates the subject of several infectious diseases encountered during pregnancy. The issue begins with an overview of maternal immunization and then reviews the most common infections considered to be particularly serious.

Infections remain a major cause of maternal and fetal morbidity and mortality worldwide. The unique maternal-fetal vascular connection in some cases serves to protect the fetus, while, in other instances, it provides a conduit for the vertical transmission of infectious agents to the vulnerable fetus. The mode of acquisition, gestational age at the time of exposure, and immunologic status of both the mother and her fetus influence disease outcome.

Each article in this issue considers the epidemiology, pathogenesis, screening, diagnosis, and treatment of an individual infectious disease with which the obstetrician should be familiar. Certain disorders, such as urinary tract infections, wound infection, and mastitis, are principal concerns to the mother, while others, such as group B streptococcal, herpes simplex, and cytomegalovirus infections, pose a risk primarily to the fetus or newborn. Other conditions, such as human immunodeficiency virus infection, viral hepatitis, suspected chorioamnionitis, mycoplasma and ureaplasma, and syphilis, can be more complex and can lead to serious morbidity for both the mother and the fetus or infant.

Dr Swamy and her very capable group of accomplished authors have provided relevant information to offer contemporary strategies on each of these subjects. Their expertise and commitment to quality care and advancement of patient safety are

Obstet Gynecol Clin N Am 41 (2014) ix–x
http://dx.doi.org/10.1016/j.ogc.2014.09.002
0889-8545/14/$ – see front matter © 2014 Published by Elsevier Inc.

obgyn.theclinics.com

exemplary. Practical evidence-based information provided herein will aid the reader in searching for timely guidelines.

William F. Rayburn, MD, MBA
Continuing Medical Education and Professional Development
University of New Mexico School of Medicine
MSC10 5580, 1 University of New Mexico
Albuquerque, NM 87131-0001, USA

E-mail address:
wrayburn@salud.unm.edu

Preface

Infectious Diseases in Pregnancy

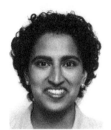

Geeta K. Swamy, MD
Editor

Human infectious diseases are caused by bacterial, viral, or fungal invasion of the body, which results in characteristic signs and symptoms of disease. The majority of infectious diseases are self-limited or readily respond to antibacterial or antiviral therapy in the healthy, immunocompetent individual. Pregnancy is a physiologically unique period when otherwise healthy women are at risk for serious infection-related complications due to the obligatory immunologic changes to allow for a diminished inflammatory response and fetal tolerance, as in the case of influenza. In addition to maternal risk, the potential for vertical or mother-to-child transmission is another infectious disease distinction of pregnancy. Vertical transmission can occur through transplacental passage, often resulting in severe congenital malformations and long-term disability, as seen with rubella and cytomegalovirus. Fetal infection can occur from ascending maternal infection of the vagina and cervix, which is often the case in chorioamnionitis. Intrapartum infection due to hematogenous spread or direct exposure during birth accounts for perinatal transmission of HIV, herpes zoster, and group B streptococcus. Postnatal transmission can occur from breastfeeding.

This issue of *Obstetrics and Gynecology Clinics of North America* provides a summary of several more common maternal-fetal-infant infectious diseases. Several experts in the field of maternal and perinatal infection have contributed to this issue to provide an overview of the up-to-date preventive strategies, screening and diagnostic methods, and treatment guidelines. While guidelines such as universal vaccination to prevent influenza during pregnancy are fairly well justified by supporting data, there is much uncertainty about the appropriate screening guidelines for conditions such as cytomegalovirus, where the lack of a proven effective treatment diminishes the value of screening. Moreover, increasing issues of antibiotic resistance and the lack of significant advancement in developing newer effective agents imply that both providers and health care facilities must follow guidelines of antimicrobial stewardship (ie, coordinated efforts to improve and measure the appropriate use of

Obstet Gynecol Clin N Am 41 (2014) xi–xii
http://dx.doi.org/10.1016/j.ogc.2014.09.001
0889-8545/14/$ – see front matter © 2014 Elsevier Inc. All rights reserved.

antimicrobials). It is our hope that this issue will aid providers in navigating these complex issues while also understanding the current state-of-the-science.

Geeta K. Swamy, MD
Department of Obstetrics and Gynecology
Division of Maternal-Fetal Medicine
Duke University School of Medicine
2608 Erwin Road, Suite 210, Durham, NC 27705, USA

E-mail address:
geeta.swamy@duke.edu

Maternal Immunization to Benefit the Mother, Fetus, and Infant

Geeta K. Swamy, MD[a],*, Rebecca Garcia-Putnam, MD[b]

KEYWORDS

- Maternal immunization • Passive immunity • Influenza • Tetanus • Pertussis

KEY POINTS

- Prevention of vaccine-preventable diseases through immunization is one of the greatest public health achievements in the United States and worldwide.
- Pregnant women are at risk for the same infections as their nonpregnant peers and, in some cases, have increased morbidity and mortality.
- Maternal immunization provides maternal, fetal (preterm birth, fetal growth restriction, and fetal demise), and infant benefit (infection during early life).
- Future research should focus on maternal vaccine immunology, efficacy and safety of maternal immunization, and the development of new vaccines against important maternal-infant pathogens.
- Obstetric providers can aid in improving vaccine coverage and overcoming barriers to maternal immunization through direct vaccine recommendation, counseling, and education.

INTRODUCTION

It is well known that the implementation of routine immunizations has had a significant impact on the health and well-being of infants, children, and adults worldwide. From 1900 to 2000 the life expectancy of a United States–born resident increased from 47.3 years to 76.8 years.[1] The great reduction and, in some cases, eradication of vaccine-preventable diseases (VPDs), along with innumerable other public health

Dr. Swamy has received past support from GlaxoSmithKline, Inc. for consultant and speaker activities which ended March 2012. Dr. Swamy has received funding from the National Institutes of Health, the Centers for Disease Control and Prevention, the American College of Obstetrics & Gynecology, and GlaxoSmithKline, Inc. to conduct vaccine-related research.
Dr. Garcia-Putnam - none.
[a] Division of Maternal-Fetal Medicine, Department of Obstetrics & Gynecology, Duke University, Durham, NC 27705, USA; [b] Department of Obstetrics & Gynecology, Duke University, Durham, NC 27705, USA
* Corresponding author. Duke Maternal-Fetal Medicine, 2608 Erwin Road, Suite 210, Durham, NC 27705.
E-mail address: geeta.swamy@duke.edu

Obstet Gynecol Clin N Am 41 (2014) 521–534
http://dx.doi.org/10.1016/j.ogc.2014.08.001
0889-8545/14/$ – see front matter © 2014 Elsevier Inc. All rights reserved.
obgyn.theclinics.com

and medical advancements, has contributed to this change, with vaccines deemed one of the greatest achievements of the decade by the Centers for Disease Control and Prevention (CDC) in 2011.[1] Polio and smallpox have been eradicated in the United States while cases of and deaths from rubella, diphtheria, tetanus, mumps, and pertussis have declined by more than 90% since the routine administration of the associated vaccines.[2] More recently the introduction of the pneumococcal vaccine has been credited with preventing more than 200,000 infections and 10,000 deaths over an 8-year period.[1]

Despite the progress made over the last century, there is still much work to be done to reduce VPDs in the United States, as routine adult vaccine coverage falls well below the Healthy People 2020 immunization goals.[3] As of 2009, there were still approximately 50,000 deaths annually from VPDs in the United States.[4] Pneumococcal disease continues to cause an estimated 30,000 cases of invasive disease, resulting in 175,000 hospitalizations for pneumonia per year.[5] Approximately 1 in 5 United States residents is infected with seasonal influenza and, depending on the circulating strain, the associated morbidity and mortality can be significant; an estimated 3000 to more than 40,000 Americans die as a result of influenza infection each year.[6]

There are now 17 VPDs covered by 14 routine, recommended vaccinations for adults.[7,8] Pregnant women are at risk for the same diseases as their nonpregnant peers and, in some cases, have increased morbidity and mortality associated with infection. For instance, pregnant women affected by seasonal and pandemic influenza viruses have higher rates of hospitalization, need for admission to the intensive care unit (ICU), pneumonia, and death.[9–15] However, pregnant women are not candidates for all vaccines, owing to the potential and theoretical risks of fetal harm. Vaccines are broadly classified into 2 categories: inactivated and live attenuated. Live attenuated vaccines contain altered pathogens that have very low virulence properties, which can replicate in the vaccinated individual and induce an immune response. Although technically possible for a live attenuated vaccine to cause a clinical infection, it is extremely uncommon and is mild in comparison with natural infection. However, given this theoretical risk of causing maternal infection and subsequent perinatal transmission, live attenuated vaccines are contraindicated in pregnancy. Inactivated vaccines contain heat-inactivated or chemically inactivated noninfectious pathogens, pathogen subunits, or toxoids, and are recommended during pregnancy based on weighing the risks and benefits of maternal-fetal exposure to the vaccine versus the exposure to infection and risks of morbidity and mortality. Because the immune response to inactivated vaccines is not cellular but rather almost entirely humoral, these vaccines tend to require multiple or booster doses to maintain adequate antibody levels over time. In addition to improving overall maternal health, there is mounting evidence that maternal immunization results in improved pregnancy outcomes and may be an effective strategy against particularly problematic VPDs during early infancy. This article describes the benefits of maternal immunization for the mother, fetus, and infant.

MATERNAL BENEFITS OF IMMUNIZATION

During pregnancy there are physiologic and immunologic changes that increase a woman's susceptibility to infection, making prevention and, thus, vaccination a highly important component of routine prenatal care. The immune response is modified to decrease inflammatory immune responses and diminish fetal rejection.[16] In addition, there is a shift from a T-helper 1 (Th1) response toward a more Th2-favored response, allowing for fetal antigen tolerance, but potentially increasing maternal vulnerability to infectious diseases.[17] This vulnerability is apparent in the increased morbidity and mortality associated with maternal influenza infection in otherwise healthy pregnant women in comparison with nonpregnant individuals. This phenomenon has been studied for decades, and was documented during the Spanish Flu pandemic of 1918 and the Asian Flu epidemic of 1959.[11,12] More recently, during the 2009 H1N1 pandemic, pregnant women were more than 4 times more likely than nonpregnant individuals to be hospitalized with influenza-related complications.[14] In addition, H1N1-infected pregnant women had higher rates of ICU admission and death than nonpregnant patients.[9,13] Seasonal influenza is also associated with more severe disease in pregnant women, who have an increased likelihood of seeking care for their symptoms and a higher rate of hospitalization because of respiratory illness.[10,14,15] Although influenza is the most well-studied VPD in pregnancy, others, such as measles and *Haemophilus influenzae*, have also been associated with significantly increased maternal morbidity and mortality.[18,19]

Given the known consequences of maternal infection, the best way to prevent many infections during pregnancy is to vaccinate pregnant women against VPDs. The CDC publishes and updates guidelines for maternal immunization.[8,20] Influenza vaccination is the most well-studied vaccine administered during pregnancy. First recommended for pregnant women in 1997, influenza vaccine is currently recommended for all pregnant women regardless of gestational age.[21] In the case of seasonal influenza, the administration of inactivated influenza vaccine has been widely studied in pregnancy, with no demonstrated safety concerns. As in nonpregnant adults, a single dose of the trivalent seasonal influenza vaccine is adequate to achieve an increase in antibody levels, in addition to seroconversion and seroprotection during pregnancy.[22–25] The H1N1 monovalent vaccine was also found to induce protective antibody levels in pregnant women.[26,27] In addition to laboratory measures of vaccine-induced protection against influenza, The Mother's Gift project demonstrated clinical efficacy of inactivated influenza vaccine. Zaman and colleagues[28] conducted a randomized controlled trial of 340 pregnant women in Bangladesh receiving either trivalent inactivated influenza or pneumococcal vaccine, and demonstrated that influenza vaccine recipients were 36% less likely to have a respiratory illness with fever than women who received the pneumococcal vaccine. Given the increased morbidity and mortality associated with influenza infection during pregnancy and the effectiveness of immunization, unless contraindicated all pregnant women who will be pregnant during the influenza season should receive the seasonal inactivated influenza vaccine.

Similar to general adult vaccination rates, maternal influenza vaccination rates have historically been suboptimal. A 2008 study found that among various adult populations recommended to receive the seasonal influenza vaccination, pregnant women had the lowest rate of immunization, at 14%.[29] However, it appears that maternal influenza vaccination rates improved after the novel H1N1 strain first circulated in 2009. During the 2009 and 2010 influenza seasons in Massachusetts, 67.5% of residents who had live births received the seasonal vaccine and 57.6% received the H1N1 vaccine.[30] Since that time vaccination rates among pregnant women have remained stable or have improved, with coverage ranging from 32% to 79%, varying widely across the country.[31] Although better than they once were, immunization rates among pregnant women can and should be improved.

Although not as well studied, it can be inferred that other vaccines known to be immunogenic and safe in pregnancy would also confer maternal benefit by reducing the likelihood of contracting infection or developing severe disease.[32] Tdap (tetanus, diphtheria, and acellular pertussis vaccine for ages 7 and older) is specifically recommended for all pregnant women after 20 weeks' gestation, regardless of previous vaccination history.[33] Although the vaccine should prevent infection in the mother, the primary indication for the Tdap recommendation is for infant benefit, reviewed in greater detail later in this article. Several vaccines are recommended for pregnant women based on the potential for maternal benefit if the risk of infection/exposure or the potential for severe/complicated illness is high. Hepatitis A, which causes an acute infection of the liver associated with jaundice, nausea, vomiting, and fever, has an associated inactivated vaccine that is recommended for all women who are at high risk of exposure, such as those traveling to endemic areas.[34] Hepatitis B, which causes acute and chronic liver inflammation and can lead to severe morbidity such as liver failure and hepatocellular carcinoma, has high rates of vertical transmission. Thus, pregnant women are routinely screened for infection, and vaccine is recommended if they are at high risk, based on sexual practices, drug use, and exposure to other hepatitis B–positive persons.[35] *Streptococcus pneumoniae* is associated with severe illness including meningitis, pneumonia, bacteremia, and acute otitis media. The introduction of pneumococcal polysaccharide 23-valent conjugate vaccine (PPSV23) has been crucial in reducing the number of cases and deaths from this disease each year in the United States.[1] Maternal vaccination with PPSV23 results in protective maternal antibody levels[36] in addition to higher neonatal antibody levels among infants born to vaccinated mothers in comparison with unvaccinated mothers.[37] Thus, vaccination should be considered for pregnant women with comorbid conditions that put them at high risk for pneumococcal disease, which include, but are not limited to, preexisting chronic heart or lung disease, diabetes mellitus, and cigarette smoking.[38] Similarly, meningococcal disease can cause serious illness, specifically meningitis, and can be prevented with a tetravalent meningococcal conjugate vaccine (MCV4). This vaccine is recommended for high-risk pregnant women, which includes, but is not limited to, those living in college or military housing, women with asplenia or complement deficiency, and those with occupational exposure.[39] All of the aforementioned vaccines, aside from influenza vaccine, are lacking strong data to support their efficacy and safety in pregnancy. However, given that these are all inactivated vaccines, the risk of fetal harm is based on theoretical concerns rather than any evidence to support adverse outcomes. In light of the severity of disease associated with these infections, the potential for maternal benefit in populations at risk is fairly high.

FETAL BENEFITS OF MATERNAL IMMUNIZATION

One commonly cited barrier to maternal vaccination is parental and provider fear of causing fetal harm.[40] Given the theoretical risks associated with antepartum vaccination, the safety of recommended vaccines in pregnancy has been looked at extensively. As discussed previously, only inactivated vaccines are considered for use during pregnancy. Moreover, inadvertent administration of live attenuated vaccines in early pregnancy, specifically measles-mumps-rubella and varicella vaccines, has never been associated with congenital infection, and thus should not be deemed as a medical indication for pregnancy termination.[41–43]

Maternal vaccination with inactivated influenza vaccine across gestation has not been associated with major birth defects, preterm birth, or fetal growth restriction.[44,45] Moreover, immunizing pregnant mothers against influenza is not only safe for the fetus but is actually associated with improved pregnancy outcomes. H1N1 infection during pregnancy has been associated with increased rates of low birth weight, preterm birth, and infant death.[46] In a subanalysis of the Mother's Gift project it was found that during the time of circulating influenza virus vaccinated mothers were less likely to have a small-for-gestational-age infant, and the mean birth weight was higher.[47] Similarly, in a study looking at more than 4000 live births in the United States, mothers who received the seasonal influenza vaccine were at lower risk of preterm birth and small-for-gestational-age infants in comparison with unvaccinated women.[48] In a large Swedish cohort study, which included more than 18,000 mother-infant pairs, influenza vaccination during pregnancy was not associated with any adverse pregnancy outcomes and was associated with decreased rates of intrauterine fetal demise, preterm birth, and low birth weight.[49] Another large European cohort study with more than 117,000 pregnancies focused on influenza vaccine safety in pregnancy, and concluded that maternal influenza vaccination significantly lowered the risk of intrauterine fetal demise.[50] These findings have important clinical implications, given the lack of effective interventions against intrauterine fetal demise and fetal growth restriction in addition to the severe morbidity and mortality associated with preterm birth and low birth weight, including respiratory distress, cerebral palsy, and the need for admission to neonatal intensive care.[51]

INFANT BENEFITS OF MATERNAL IMMUNIZATION

Early infant immunity is fairly immature, complex, and highly dependent on maternal immunity because of the phenomenon of transplacental transfer of maternal antibodies to the developing fetus. First studied in the 1800s, it was observed that infants born to mothers who had survived pertussis were less likely to contract pertussis early in life.[52] In the 1970s, antibody levels of women colonized with group B *Streptococcus* (GBS) were found to correlate with neonatal infection, such that infants of mothers with lower antibody titers were more likely to develop GBS infection.[53] Later the mechanism was investigated, and in vitro studies demonstrated that there is a preferential transport of maternally derived immunoglobulin G (IgG) from the maternal to the fetal side of the human placenta.[54] Although the mechanism of IgG transport across the placenta is not fully understood, studies examining the timing of IgG transport have found that fetal IgG levels increase with increasing gestational age, perhaps indicating that there are particular changes in placental physiology or IgG receptor expression that allow for greater penetration of the antibody.[55] Specifically, the FcRn receptor has been associated with preferential transport of IgG subclasses 1 and 3.[52,55] Studies have also confirmed that vaccine-induced IgG behaves similarly to disease-induced IgG, with transplacental transfer observed after maternal *Haemophilus influenzae* and pneumococcal vaccination.[56,57] Together these findings demonstrate that maternal IgG crosses the placenta and provides effective neonatal protection against viral and bacterial infections early in life.

Based on documented transplacental antibody transfer and the high susceptibility to infection during the first months of life, maternal immunization has been posed as a means of boosting passive immunity by achieving higher maternal and fetal/neonatal antibody levels against VPDs. This scenario is particularly relevant for VPDs that pose significant morbidity and mortality for young infants and do not have any other effective means of prevention such as a neonatal vaccine. Current data support the infant benefits of maternal immunization against influenza, tetanus, and pertussis.[28,32,33,58] Influenza infection in young infants is associated with substantial morbidity, including dehydration, pneumonia, and encephalopathy requiring hospitalization.[46,59,60] Influenza infection can also result in infant death, with 16 of the 115 (14%) pediatric influenza deaths during the 2010-2011 season occurring in infants younger than 6 months.[61] There is currently no licensed influenza vaccine capable of producing an immunogenic response in infants younger than 6 months, leaving this group of children unprotected during an extremely vulnerable period for developing severe illness.[62] The Mother's Gift project was able to demonstrate that maternal vaccination conferred infant protection from influenza, and specifically showed a 63% reduction in laboratory-proven influenza and a 29% reduction in febrile illness in infants born to vaccinated mothers when compared with those born to unvaccinated mothers.[28] Furthermore, it has been demonstrated that infants of vaccinated mothers maintain protective antibody levels against influenza A strains for as long as 10 weeks, and at 20 weeks have significantly higher levels than infants born to unvaccinated mothers.[25] In addition, a United States–based study showed that maternal influenza vaccination was 91.5% effective at preventing influenza-related hospitalization in infants younger than 6 months.[63] Of note, infant antibody levels may vary depending on timing of maternal vaccination, such that third-trimester vaccination leads to higher maternal and cord blood titers in comparison with first- or second-trimester vaccination.[64]

The World Health Organization (WHO) maternal and neonatal tetanus elimination program is an ongoing project to vaccinate mothers to reduce rates of neonatal tetanus in developing countries.[58] Tetanus is among the most lethal consequences of the unsanitary birth practices that occur in many areas with limited health care resources, and in 1988 accounted for as many as 787,000 neonatal deaths worldwide. The strategy for vaccine administration targets women of reproductive age and, once they become pregnant, they begin the vaccine schedule that includes 2 tetanus vaccine doses 1 month apart during the initial pregnancy, a third dose 6 months later, and additional doses in each subsequent pregnancy for a total of 5 doses. This program has demonstrated that even multiple doses of tetanus vaccine are safe, with more than 17 million women having received at least 2 doses during pregnancy.[65] This initiative has been extremely successful, lowering the estimated number of tetanus-related neonatal deaths by 93% over a 20-year period, and demonstrating that a model of maternal immunization for neonatal disease prevention is feasible on a large scale.[58]

Pertussis is another infection that can cause severe respiratory disease and mortality in young infants. Unlike the presentation in older children or adults, neonatal infection can progress from mild symptoms, such as low-grade fever, cough, or rhinorrhea, to severe respiratory distress very quickly.[66] The currently recommended schedule for pediatric DTaP (similar to Tdap but for children $\leq$7 years) administration begins at 2 months of age followed by booster doses at 4, 6, and 15 to 18 months, and 4 to 6 years of age.[67] Unfortunately, this leaves the most vulnerable group, young infants, unprotected against pertussis until about 4 months of age. Cortese and colleagues[68] studied infants until 6 months of age and found that a significant decrease in hospitalization for pertussis did not occur until after administration of 2 doses of DTaP. Similarly to influenza vaccine, infants do not seem to mount an adequate response to vaccination against pertussis during the first few months of life. Halasa and colleagues[69] performed a randomized trial comparing DTaP-induced antibody responses in infants following the recommended vaccination schedule, plus an additional dose in the first 14 days of life to the recommended vaccination schedule only. Although there were no safety concerns following a "birth" dose of DTaP, the antibody response was actually reduced in the group who received the additional birth dose, raising concerns about efficacy and even potential harm. Recent vaccine studies using a baboon model of pertussis infection suggest that neonatal vaccination could improve immunity, necessitating the need for further research.[70]

Over the past few years the recommendations for Tdap administration in pregnant and postpartum women have changed considerably. Most recently, in October 2012 the CDC's Advisory Committee on Immunization Practice (ACIP) committee revised the recommended schedule for maternal vaccination, stating that all pregnant women, regardless of previous Tdap immunization, should be vaccinated between 27 and 36 weeks' gestation[33]; this was a change from prior efforts that focused on hospital-based postpartum vaccination.[71,72] The greatly increased incidence of pertussis and infant deaths in the United States in 2012 triggered this swift and aggressive recommendation, which was quickly adopted by the American College of Obstetrics and Gynecology and the American Academy of Pediatricians.[73,74]

There is still a tremendous amount of work to be done to optimize maternal Tdap administration. The current timing of administration, during the third trimester, is recommended based on the known increased rate of transplacental antibody transfer later in gestation,[75] rather than on data showing that this strategy is the most effective. One small study did demonstrate that women vaccinated intrapartum, compared with those vaccinated preconception, tend to have higher cord blood antibody titers at delivery.[76] However, this study was limited by small sample size and lack of statistical significance, such that it is unclear if these results would be reproduced with a larger sample size. Furthermore, immunity wanes over time such that maternally derived antibodies against pertussis decline to undetectable levels in the infant by 2 months of age, which raises questions regarding the usefulness of maternal vaccination in preventing infantile pertussis and the robustness of the immune response to the acellular pertussis vaccine.[77–79] Witt and colleagues[80] demonstrated that nonpregnant adults who received the acellular vaccine had a significantly higher risk of contracting pertussis in comparison with those who received the whole cell vaccine. In addition, there are concerns that circulating maternal antibodies in the infant may interfere with the innate immune response to routine infant vaccination, such as the DTaP series. At present the evidence for this phenomenon is conflicting. One study did demonstrate that infants of Tdap-vaccinated mothers had a less robust primary response to the DTaP series than those born to unvaccinated mothers,[81] while a recent study showed no significant difference in the infant immune response to DTaP up to 13 months of age when comparing by maternal vaccination status.[32] Although more work is needed to clarify the risks and benefits of maternal Tdap vaccination, the theoretical benefit to the infant is great and likely outweighs the risks. Furthermore, Tdap vaccine in pregnancy seems to be safe and is not associated with any adverse pregnancy outcomes.[8,32] Given the lack of an effective neonatal vaccine and the rising incidence of pertussis in the United States over the last few decades, obstetric providers are urged to follow the current CDC recommendation of third-trimester Tdap vaccination for all pregnant women, regardless of prior receipt, as a means of reducing neonatal pertussis.[8,33]

Given the many infectious diseases that affect both mothers and infants, there are several candidate pathogens that are being targeted for maternal-fetal-infant vaccine development. GBS is a bacterium that colonizes the vagina in a subset of pregnant women and can cause severe neonatal disease including sepsis, meningitis, and death. Although neonatal GBS rates declined significantly following the implementation of universal maternal screening for and intrapartum treatment of known GBS infection, the incidence of neonatal GBS has been stagnant in recent years, and a vaccine may be the next step in lowering the disease burden.[82,83] A candidate vaccine has been developed, and preliminary trials have begun to assess acceptability and uptake in addition to safety and immunogenicity.[84–88] Cost-effectiveness trials have shown that a GBS vaccine would not only greatly reduce neonatal risk, but in a South African population would be cost-effective by WHO standards.[89] Another very common infection in young infants is respiratory syncytial virus (RSV), which causes significant lower respiratory tract disease that frequently requires hospitalization in infants younger than 6 months.[90] There are projects ongoing to determine the feasibility of a maternal vaccination to provide passive immunity.[91–94] These efforts are supported by data showing that maternal RSV antibodies are effective in preventing RSV disease in young, RSV-naïve infants.[92,95–97]

SUMMARY

Prevention of VPDs through immunization is one of the greatest public health achievements in the United States and worldwide. Immunizing women during pregnancy with recommended vaccines provides direct maternal benefit. In addition, maternal immunization has potential fetal benefits by preventing adverse pregnancy outcomes (preterm birth, fetal growth restriction, and fetal demise), and potential infant benefit by preventing infection during early life. Research should continue to focus on maternal vaccine immunology, efficacy, and safety of current vaccines, and the development of new vaccines against important maternal-infant pathogens, to elucidate optimal maternal immunization strategies that will maximize maternal and infant benefit. Vaccine uptake varies greatly across the country and has been shown to be highly influenced by provider recommendation, implying that simply recommending the vaccine is the first step in improving vaccine uptake.[30,40,98] Public health officials and obstetrics and gynecology (ObGyn) providers can help to overcome barriers to immunization, such as safety and financial concerns, through counseling and education. Previous maternal vaccine initiatives, including screening for rubella immunity and immunization for Rh disease, demonstrate that the ObGyn community is capable of making changes in vaccine uptake.[99,100] The importance of improving maternal immunization rates cannot be understated. The benefits of vaccination are 3-fold: (1) protecting the mother from antepartum infection; (2) reducing poor pregnancy and fetal outcomes; and (3) providing immunity for neonates during the vulnerable first few months of life.

REFERENCES

1. Centers for Disease Control and Prevention. Ten great public health achievements—United States, 2001-2010. MMWR Morb Mortal Wkly Rep 2011;60(19): 619–23.
2. Roush SW, Murphy TV. Historical comparisons of morbidity and mortality for vaccine-preventable diseases in the United States. JAMA 2007;298(18): 2155–63.
3. 2020 Topics and objectives: immunizations and infectious diseases. 2014. Available at: http://www.healthypeople.gov/2020/topicsobjectives2020/objectiveslist. aspx?topicId=23. Accessed January 2, 2014.
4. Facts about adult immunization. 2009. Available at: http://www.nfid.org/ publications/factsheets/adultfact.pdf. Accessed December 30, 2013.
5. Pneumococcal disease. 2014. Available at: http://www.adultvaccination.com/ vpd/pneumococcal. Accessed January 3, 2014.
6. Influenza (Flu). 2014. Available at: http://www.adultvaccination.com/vpd/influenza. Accessed May 30, 2014.
7. National Center for Immunization and Respiratory Diseases. General recommendations on immunization - recommendations of the Advisory Committee on Immunization Practices (ACIP). MMWR Recomm Rep 2011;60(2):1–64.
8. Recommended adult immunization schedule. 2014. Available at: http://www. cdc.gov/vaccines/schedules/downloads/adult/adult-combined-schedule.pdf. Accessed May 29, 2014.

9. Louie JK, Acosta M, Jamieson DJ, et al. Severe 2009 H1N1 influenza in pregnant and postpartum women in California. N Engl J Med 2010;362(1):27–35.
10. Neuzil KM, Reed GW, Mitchel EF, et al. Impact of influenza on acute cardiopulmonary hospitalizations in pregnant women. Am J Epidemiol 1998;148(11): 1094–102.
11. Harris JW. Influenza occurring in pregnant women: a statistical study of thirteen hundred and fifty cases. JAMA 1919;72:978–80.
12. Freeman DW, Barno A. Deaths from Asian influenza associated with pregnancy. Am J Obstet Gynecol 1959;78:1172–5.
13. Siston AM, Rasmussen SA, Honein MA, et al. Pandemic 2009 influenza A(H1N1) virus illness among pregnant women in the United States. JAMA 2010;303(15): 1517–25.
14. Jamieson DJ, Honeine MA, Rasmussen SA, et al. H1N1 2009 influenza virus infection during pregnancy in the USA. Lancet 2009;374(9688):451–8.
15. Dodds L, McNeil SA, Fell DB, et al. Impact of influenza exposure on rates of hospital admissions and physician visits because of respiratory illness among pregnant women. CMAJ 2007;176(4):463–8.
16. Raghupathy R. Th1-type immunity is incompatible with successful pregnancy. Immunol Today 1997;18(10):478–82.
17. Robinson DP, Klein SL. Pregnancy and pregnancy-associated hormones alter immune responses and disease pathogenesis. Horm Behav 2012;62(3):263–71.
18. Ogbuanu IU, Zeko S, Chu SY, et al. Maternal, fetal, and neonatal outcomes associated with measles during pregnancy: Namibia, 2009-2010. Clin Infect Dis 2014;58(8):1086–92.
19. Collins S, Ramsay M, Slack MP, et al. Risk of invasive *Haemophilus influenzae* infection during pregnancy and association with adverse fetal outcomes. JAMA 2014;311(11):1125–32.
20. Swamy GK, Garcia-Putnam R. Vaccine-preventable diseases in pregnancy. Am J Perinatol 2013;30(2):89–97.
21. Prevention and control of influenza: recommendations of the Advisory Committee on Immunization Practices (ACIP). MMWR Recomm Rep 1997;46(RR-9):1–25.
22. Jackson LA, Patel SM, Swamy GK, et al. Immunogenicity of an inactivated monovalent 2009 H1N1 influenza vaccine in pregnant women. J Infect Dis 2011;204(6):854–63.
23. Schlaudecker EP, McNeal MM, Dodd CN, et al. Pregnancy modifies the antibody response to trivalent influenza immunization. J Infect Dis 2012;206(11): 1670–3.
24. Englund JA, Mbawuike IN, Hammill H, et al. Maternal immunization with influenza or tetanus toxoid vaccine for passive antibody protection in young infants. J Infect Dis 1993;168(3):647–56.
25. Steinhoff MC, Omer SB, Roy E, et al. Influenza immunization in pregnancy—antibody responses in mothers and infants. N Engl J Med 2010;362(17):1644–6.
26. Tsatsaris V, Capitant C, Schmitz T, et al. Maternal immune response and neonatal seroprotection from a single dose of a monovalent nonadjuvanted 2009 influenza A(H1N1) vaccine: a single-group trial. Ann Intern Med 2011; 155(11):733–41.
27. Fisher BM, Van Bockern J, Hart J, et al. Pandemic influenza A H1N1 2009 infection versus vaccination: a cohort study comparing immune responses in pregnancy. PLoS One 2012;7(3):e33048.
28. Zaman K, Roy E, Arifeen SE, et al. Effectiveness of maternal influenza immunization in mothers and infants. N Engl J Med 2008;359(15):1555–64.

29. Lu P, Bridges CB, Euler GL, et al. Influenza vaccination of recommended adult populations, U.S., 1989-2005. Vaccine 2008;26(14):1786–93.

30. Centers for Disease Control and Prevention (CDC). Influenza vaccination among pregnant women–Massachusetts, 2009-2010. MMWR Morb Mortal Wkly Rep 2013;62(43):854–7.

31. Centers for Disease Control and Prevention (CDC). Seasonal influenza vaccination coverage among women who delivered a live-born infant - 21 states and New York City, 2009-10 and 2010-11 influenza seasons. MMWR Morb Mortal Wkly Rep 2013;62(49):1001–4.

32. Munoz FM, Bond NH, Maccato M, et al. Safety and immunogenicity of tetanus diphtheria and acellular pertussis (Tdap) immunization during pregnancy in mothers and infants: a randomized clinical trial. JAMA 2014; 311(17):1760–9.

33. Centers for Disease Control and Prevention (CDC). Updated recommendations for use of tetanus toxoid, reduced diphtheria toxoid, and acellular pertussis vaccine (Tdap) in pregnant women–Advisory Committee on Immunization Practices (ACIP), 2012. MMWR Morb Mortal Wkly Rep 2013;62(7):131–5.

34. Fiore AE, Wasley A, Bell BP. Prevention of hepatitis A through active or passive immunization: recommendations of the Advisory Committee on Immunization Practices (ACIP). MMWR Recomm Rep 2006;55(RR-7):1–23.

35. Mast EE, Weinbaum CM, Fiore AE, et al. A comprehensive immunization strategy to eliminate transmission of hepatitis B virus infection in the United States: recommendations of the Advisory Committee on Immunization Practices (ACIP) Part II: immunization of adults [quiz: CE1–4]. MMWR Recomm Rep 2006; 55(RR-16):1–33.

36. Schlaudecker EP, Steinhoff MC, Omer SB, et al. Antibody persistence in mothers one year after pneumococcal immunization in pregnancy. Vaccine 2012;30(34): 5063–6.

37. Shahid NS, Steinhoff MC, Hoque SS, et al. Serum, breast milk, and infant antibody after maternal immunisation with pneumococcal vaccine. Lancet 1995; 346(8985):1252–7.

38. Centers for Disease Control and Prevention (CDC), Advisory Committee on Immunization Practices. Updated recommendations for prevention of invasive pneumococcal disease among adults using the 23-valent pneumococcal polysaccharide vaccine (PPSV23). MMWR Morb Mortal Wkly Rep 2010;59(34): 1102–6.

39. Bilukha OO, Rosenstein N. Prevention and control of meningococcal disease. Recommendations of the Advisory Committee on Immunization Practices (ACIP). MMWR Recomm Rep 2005;54(RR-7):1–21.

40. Panda B, Stiller R, Panda A. Influenza vaccination during pregnancy and factors for lacking compliance with current CDC guidelines. J Matern Fetal Neonatal Med 2011;24(3):402–6.

41. Centers for Disease Control and Prevention (CDC). Revised ACIP recommendation for avoiding pregnancy after receiving a rubella-containing vaccine. MMWR Morb Mortal Wkly Rep 2001;50(49):1117.

42. Marin M, Guris D, Chaves SS, et al. Prevention of varicella: recommendations of the Advisory Committee on Immunization Practices (ACIP). MMWR Recomm Rep 2007;56(RR-4):1–40.

43. Merck pregnancy registries: Varicella zoster virus-containing vaccines. 2014. Available at: http://www.merckpregnancyregistries.com/varivax.html. Accessed January 3, 2014.

44. Pasternak B, Svanstrom H, Molgaard-Nielsen D, et al. Risk of adverse fetal outcomes following administration of a pandemic influenza A(H1N1) vaccine during pregnancy. JAMA 2012;308(2):165–74.
45. Lin SY, Wu ET, Lin CH, et al. The safety and immunogenicity of trivalent inactivated influenza vaccination: a study of maternal-cord blood pairs in Taiwan. PLoS One 2013;8(6):e62983.
46. Doyle TJ, Goodin K, Hamilton JJ. Maternal and neonatal outcomes among pregnant women with 2009 pandemic influenza A(H1N1) illness in Florida, 2009–2010: a population-based cohort study. PLoS One 2013;8(10):e79040.
47. Steinhoff MC, Omer SB. A review of fetal and infant protection associated with antenatal influenza immunization. Am J Obstet Gynecol 2012;207(3 Suppl): S21–7.
48. Omer SB, Goodman D, Steinhoff MC, et al. Maternal influenza immunization and reduced likelihood of prematurity and small for gestational age births: a retrospective cohort study. PLoS Med 2011;8(5):e1000441.
49. Kallen B, Olausson PO. Vaccination against H1N1 influenza with Pandemrix((R)) during pregnancy and delivery outcome: a Swedish register study. BJOG 2012; 119(13):1583–90.
50. Haberg SE, Trogstad L, Gunnes N, et al. Risk of fetal death after pandemic influenza virus infection or vaccination. N Engl J Med 2013;368(4):333–40.
51. Behrman RE, Butler AS, editors. Preterm birth: causes, consequences, and prevention. Washington, DC: National Academy of Sciences; 2007.
52. Englund JA. The influence of maternal immunization on infant immune responses. J Comp Pathol 2007;137(Suppl 1):S16–9.
53. Baker CJ, Kasper DL. Correlation of maternal antibody deficiency with susceptibility to neonatal group B streptococcal infection. N Engl J Med 1976;294(14): 753–6.
54. Malek A. Ex vivo human placenta models: transport of immunoglobulin G and its subclasses. Vaccine 2003;21(24):3362–4.
55. Simister NE. Placental transport of immunoglobulin G. Vaccine 2003;21(24): 3365–9.
56. Englund JA, Glezen WP, Turner C, et al. Transplacental antibody transfer following maternal immunization with polysaccharide and conjugate Haemophilus influenzae type b vaccines. J Infect Dis 1995;171(1):99–105.
57. Munoz FM, Englund JA, Cheesman CC, et al. Maternal immunization with pneumococcal polysaccharide vaccine in the third trimester of gestation. Vaccine 2001;20(5–6):826–37.
58. Maternal and Neonatal Tetanus (MNT) elimination. 2014. Available at: http://www.who.int/immunization/diseases/MNTE_initiative/en/. Accessed June 1, 2014.
59. Poehling KA, Edwards KM, Weinberg GA, et al. The underrecognized burden of influenza in young children. N Engl J Med 2006;355(1):31–40.
60. Protecting against influenza (Flu): advice for caregivers of children less than 6 months old. 2013. Available at: http://www.cdc.gov/flu/protect/infantcare.htm. Accessed June 1, 2014.
61. Centers for Disease Control and Prevention (CDC). Influenza-associated pediatric deaths–United States, September 2010-August 2011. MMWR Morb Mortal Wkly Rep 2011;60(36):1233–8.
62. Centers for Disease Control and Prevention (CDC). Prevention and control of seasonal influenza with vaccines. Recommendations of the Advisory Committee on Immunization Practices–United States, 2013-2014. MMWR Recomm Rep 2013;62(RR-07):1–43.

63. Benowitz I, Esposito DB, Gracey KD, et al. Influenza vaccine given to pregnant women reduces hospitalization due to influenza in their infants. Clin Infect Dis 2010;51(12):1355–61.
64. Garcia-Putnam R, Heine RP, Walter EB, et al. Effect of timing of influenza vaccination in pregnancy on maternal and cord blood antibody titers 2013: abstract: Society for Maternal Fetal Medicine Conference. San Francisco, February 16, 2013.
65. Vandelaer J, Birmingham M, Gasse F, et al. Tetanus in developing countries: an update on the maternal and neonatal tetanus elimination initiative. Vaccine 2003; 21(24):3442–5.
66. Nieves DJ, Singh J, Ashouri N, et al. Clinical and laboratory features of pertussis in infants at the onset of a California epidemic. J Pediatr 2011;159(6):1044–6.
67. Akinsanya-Beysolow I. Advisory Committee on Immunization Practices recommended immunization schedules for persons aged 0 through 18 years - United States, 2014. MMWR Morb Mortal Wkly Rep 2014;63(5):108–9.
68. Cortese MM, Baughman AL, Zhang R, et al. Pertussis hospitalizations among infants in the United States, 1993 to 2004. Pediatrics 2008;121(3):484–92.
69. Halasa NB, O'Shea A, Shi JR, et al. Poor immune responses to a birth dose of diphtheria, tetanus, and acellular pertussis vaccine. J Pediatr 2008;153(3): 327–32.
70. Warfel JM, Papin JF, Wolf RF, et al. Maternal and neonatal vaccination protects newborn baboons from pertussis infection. J Infect Dis 2014;210(4):604–10.
71. Meeting of the Advisory Committee on Immunization Practices (ACIP) summary report. Available at: http://www.cdc.gov/vaccines/acip/meetings/minutes-archive. html. Accessed May 29, 2014.
72. CDC Advisory Committee for immunization practices recommends Tdap immunization for pregnant women. 2012. Available at: http://www.cdc.gov/media/ releases/2012/a1024_Tdap_immunization.html. Accessed January 3, 2014.
73. CDC. 2012 final pertussis surveillance report. 2012. Available at: http://www. cdc.gov/pertussis/downloads/pertuss-surv-report-2012.pdf. Accessed June 1, 2014.
74. ACOG Committee Opinion No. 566: update on immunization and pregnancy: tetanus, diphtheria, and pertussis vaccination. Obstet Gynecol 2013;121(6): 1411–4.
75. Malek A, Sager R, Kuhn P, et al. Evolution of maternofetal transport of immunoglobulins during human pregnancy. Am J Reprod Immunol 1996;36(5):248–55.
76. Healy CM, Rench MA, Baker CJ. Importance of timing of maternal combined tetanus, diphtheria, and acellular pertussis (Tdap) immunization and protection of young infants. Clin Infect Dis 2013;56(4):539–44.
77. Healy CM, Munoz FM, Rench MA, et al. Prevalence of pertussis antibodies in maternal delivery, cord, and infant serum. J Infect Dis 2004;190(2):335–40.
78. Gall SA. Prevention of pertussis, tetanus, and diphtheria among pregnant, postpartum women, and infants. Clin Obstet Gynecol 2012;55(2):498–509.
79. Gall SA, Myers J, Pichichero M. Maternal immunization with tetanus-diphtheria-pertussis vaccine: effect on maternal and neonatal serum antibody levels. Am J Obstet Gynecol 2011;204(4):334.e1–5.
80. Witt MA, Arias L, Katz PH, et al. Reduced risk of pertussis among persons ever vaccinated with whole cell pertussis vaccine compared to recipients of acellular pertussis vaccines in a large US cohort. Clin Infect Dis 2013;56(9):1248–54.
81. Hardy-Fairbanks AJ, Pan SJ, Decker MD, et al. Immune responses in infants whose mothers received Tdap vaccine during pregnancy. Pediatr Infect Dis J 2013;32(11):1257–60.

82. Chen VL, Avci FY, Kasper DL. A maternal vaccine against group B Strepto-coccus: past, present, and future. Vaccine 2013;31(Suppl 4):D13–9.
83. Verani JR, McGee L, Schrag SJ. Prevention of perinatal group B streptococcal disease–revised guidelines from CDC, 2010. MMWR Recomm Rep 2010; 59(RR-10):1–36.
84. Ault KA, Hurwitz JA, Zimet GD, et al. The acceptability of a novel group B strep-tococcus vaccine in pregnant women. Obstet Gynecol 2014;123(Suppl 1): 131S–2S.
85. Regan JA, Klebanoff MA, Nugent RP. The epidemiology of group B strepto-coccal colonization in pregnancy. Vaginal Infections and Prematurity Study Group. Obstet Gynecol 1991;77(4):604–10.
86. Safety and immunogenicity of a trivalent group B streptococcus vaccine in health pregnant women. Ongoing Novartis Vaccine trial. 2014. Available at: https://clinicaltrials.gov/ct2/show/NCT02046148?term=novartis+and+gbs+ vaccine&rank=1. Accessed June 2, 2014.
87. Safety and immunogenicity of a Group B streptococcus vaccine in non preg-nant and pregnant women 18–40 years of age. Ongoing Novartis Vaccine trial. 2014. Available at: https://clinicaltrials.gov/ct2/show/study/NCT01193920? term=novartis+and+gbs+vaccine&rank=6&sect=X30156. Accessed June 2, 2014.
88. Immune response induced by a vaccine against group B streptococcus and safety in pregnant women and their offspring. 2014. Available at: https:// clinicaltrials.gov/ct2/show/NCT01446289?term=novartis+and+gbs+vaccine& rank=10. Accessed June 2, 2014.
89. Kim SY, Russell LB, Park J, et al. Cost-effectiveness of a potential group B strep-tococcal vaccine program for pregnant women in South Africa. Vaccine 2014; 32(17):1954–63.
90. Hall CB, Weinberg GA, Iwane MK, et al. The burden of respiratory syncytial virus infection in young children. N Engl J Med 2009;360(6):588–98.
91. Lindsey B, Kampmann B, Jones C. Maternal immunization as a strategy to decrease susceptibility to infection in newborn infants. Curr Opin Infect Dis 2013;26(3):248–53.
92. Kaaijk P, Luytjes W, Rots NY. Vaccination against RSV: is maternal vaccination a good alternative to other approaches? Hum Vaccin Immunother 2013;9(6): 1263–7.
93. Anderson LJ, Dormitzer PR, Nokes DJ, et al. Strategic priorities for respira-tory syncytial virus (RSV) vaccine development. Vaccine 2013;31(Suppl 2): B209–15.
94. RSV F Dose-ranging study in women. 2013. Available at: http://clinicaltrials.gov/ ct2/show/NCT01960686?term=rsv+and+novavax&rank=4. Accessed June 2, 2014.
95. Groothuis JR, Hoopes JM, Jessie VG. Prevention of serious respiratory syncytial virus-related illness. I: disease pathogenesis and early attempts at prevention. Adv Ther 2011;28(2):91–109.
96. Ogilvie MM, Vathenen AS, Radford M, et al. Maternal antibody and respiratory syncytial virus infection in infancy. J Med Virol 1981;7(4):263–71.
97. Stensballe LG, Ravn H, Kristensen K, et al. Seasonal variation of maternally derived respiratory syncytial virus antibodies and association with infant hospi-talizations for respiratory syncytial virus. J Pediatr 2009;154(2):296–8.
98. Kuehn BM. Mothers take physicians' advice on vaccines. JAMA 2010;304(23): 2577–8.

99. McLean HQ, Fiebelkorn AP, Temte JL, et al. Prevention of measles, rubella, congenital rubella syndrome, and mumps, 2013: summary recommendations of the Advisory Committee on Immunization Practices (ACIP). MMWR Recomm Rep 2013;62(RR-04):1–34.
100. Crowther C, Middleton P. Anti-D administration after childbirth for preventing Rhesus alloimmunisation. Cochrane Database Syst Rev 2000;(2):CD000021.

Prevention and Management of Influenza in Pregnancy

Richard H. Beigi, MD, MSc[a,b,*]

KEYWORDS

- Influenza • Pregnancy • Influenza vaccine

KEY POINTS

- Pregnancy increases the risk for severe disease, hospitalization, and mortality from influenza infection.
- In addition to negative effects on the mother, influenza infection is associated with untoward pregnancy outcomes such as preterm birth and small-for-gestational-age infants.
- Immunization with the inactivated influenza vaccine is the most effective way to prevent influenza infection, and all pregnant women lacking contraindication should be immunized against influenza.
- Antiviral medications have been found to reduce the risk of influenza infection after exposure and the severity and duration of infection among those infected. Obstetric providers should have a low threshold for use of the neuraminidase inhibitors for prevention and treatment of influenza in pregnancy.

INTRODUCTION AND EPIDEMIOLOGY

Influenza has been known to cause recurrent worldwide epidemics of febrile respiratory disease for at least 400 years. In this approximate period, records indicate that we have experienced at least 31 influenza pandemics. The most severe recorded influenza pandemic was the 1918 to 1919 "Spanish flu," with estimates of global mortality of at least 20 million. Looking specifically at the effects of the Spanish flu in the United

The author has nothing to disclose.
[a] Division of Obstetric Specialties, Department of Obstetrics, Gynecology, Reproductive Sciences, Magee-Womens Hospital of the University of Pittsburgh School of Medicine and Medical Center, 300 Halket Street, Room # 2326, Pittsburgh, PA 15213, USA; [b] Division of Reproductive Infectious Diseases and Immunology, Department of Obstetrics, Gynecology, Reproductive Sciences, Magee-Womens Hospital of the University of Pittsburgh School of Medicine and Medical Center, 300 Halket Street, Room # 2326, Pittsburgh, PA 15213, USA
* Department of Obstetrics, Gynecology, Reproductive Sciences, Magee-Womens Hospital, 300 Halket Street, Room # 2326, Pittsburgh, PA 15213.
E-mail address: rbeigi@mail.magee.edu

Obstet Gynecol Clin N Am 41 (2014) 535–546
http://dx.doi.org/10.1016/j.ogc.2014.08.002
0889-8545/14/$ – see front matter © 2014 Elsevier Inc. All rights reserved.

States, more than 500,000 attributable deaths were recorded in the United States during a span of 1.5 years.[1]

Influenza is an ongoing source of human morbidity and mortality. The latest Centers for Disease Control and Prevention (CDC) estimates suggest that domestic annual attributable mortality from seasonal influenza infection alone varies from 3000 to more than 49,000 per year, depending on strain specifics and additional variables.[2] In addition to mortality, the estimated 25 to 50 million cases of domestic seasonal influenza are responsible for millions of days of illness with work and school absenteeism and more than 200,000 annual influenza-related hospitalizations.[3] The combined direct medical costs and lost income related to seasonal influenza disease are significant at an estimated $26.8 billion annually in the United States.[4] Importantly, pregnancy is one of a few recognized clinical conditions that increase risk of hospitalization, serious complications, and death from influenza infection.

Influenza viruses are enveloped, single-stranded, RNA viruses in the Orthomyxoviridae family. Influenza viruses are further divided into influenza virus types A, B, and C based on particular antigenic profiles. Although all 3 influenza types have been implicated in human disease, influenza A and B strains cause most human infections. Thus, influenza A and B are the primary focus of clinical prevention and treatment efforts on a yearly basis. Additionally, thus far, only type A has been associated with the occasional influenza pandemic. Additional subdivision into serotypes is done based on their surface proteins, hemagglutinin (HA) and neuraminidase (NA). Currently, 16 different HA glycoproteins (H1–H16) and 9 NA serotypes (N1–N9) have been identified. This large number of strains contributes to the well-known influenza strain variability.

Importantly, these surface glycoproteins are important for viral entry into and exit from epithelial cells lining the human respiratory tract and are the basis of the H and N naming designations for all influenza strains (ie, H1N1 or H3N2).[1] Briefly, the HA protein mediates binding to extracellular receptors, facilitating fusion of viral and host membranes, and the NA protein acts on sialic acid residues on the surface of host cells to direct release of newly synthesized viral particles.[1,5] These viral particles go on to infect new host cells, thus, propagating the systemic infection. Respectively, these 2 proteins are the current pharmacologic targets of the 2 classes of anti-influenza medications, the adamantanes (eg, amantadine and rimantadine) and neuraminidase inhibitors (eg, oseltamivir and zanamivir). Since 2009, the adamantanes are no longer recommended for general use because of concerns about large-scale resistance among circulating influenza viruses.[6]

Influenza is also appreciated for its ongoing and naturally occurring viral alterations and mutations. These ongoing viral changes are what generate the altered antigenic characteristics, in turn, driving the necessity of yearly alterations to vaccine composition (antigenic drift). Similar antigenic differences, yet more dramatic and fundamental, are what give rise to the occasional influenza pandemic (antigenic shift). Antigenic drift is the perpetually ongoing process of modest antigenic alterations producing antigenic structures different enough for immune memory evasion. This occurs in all influenza subtypes and is responsible for yearly epidemics and the concomitant need for yearly considerations of the relevance and potential disease prevention impact of vaccine formulations. Antigenic shift is a much rarer occurrence (but nevertheless part of the natural influenza lifecycle) when 2 or more different influenza strains combine to produce a novel antigenic structure that has negligible recognition within the population. This process is currently known to occur only in influenza A viruses and happens approximately once every 20 to 30 years. This rare, yet ongoing occurrence is what produces the occasional influenza pandemic, such as the 2009 H1N1 pandemic. These "new" characteristics of the viral surface structure generated from antigenic shift produce a virus that has large population susceptibility with concomitant wide-spread disease typical of influenza pandemics.[1,7,8]

Epidemic influenza produces respiratory disease in a typically seasonal pattern, mostly from October through May (typically peaks in the early winter months) in northern hemisphere climates. In the southern hemispheres, this pattern is reversed; epidemic influenza disease is noted most frequently in May through October. Annual infection rates fluctuate based on strain virulence and background population immunity. It is thought that, in general, most yearly epidemics infect approximately 10% to 20% of the population. There are little data specifically focusing on epidemiology of infection in pregnant women, and there is no current evidence to suggest that pregnancy alters susceptibility to contracting influenza. Prevalence of influenza infection during pregnancy appears to be similar to that of the general population.[8,9] However, as is noted in the sections that follow, much historical data along with recent data from the 2009 pandemic clearly show that pregnant women suffer from increased risks of complications and mortality from influenza. This finding is most notable when considering the documented experiences from the occasional 20th and 21st century influenza pandemics.[8,10–14]

CLINICAL CHARACTERISTICS

Influenza infection is primarily transmitted person-to-person via large droplets generated by coughing and sneezing from an already infected (and often incubating) person. In addition to droplet spread, transmission is also possible by contact, either directly between an infected individual and a susceptible host or via passive transfer of virus to a susceptible host via an intermediate object (ie, contaminated hands or inanimate objects). Airborne transmission of aerosolized microorganisms or airborne droplet nuclei among persons not in close contact seems less likely.[1]

The incubation period for influenza is from 1 to 4 days and is followed by a relatively acute onset of fever, chills, nonproductive cough, nasal congestion, headache, sore throat, and constitutional symptoms such as fatigue and malaise. Most patients with influenza have a predominance of systemic symptoms along with the upper respiratory symptoms. This combination of findings can help differentiate influenza from other common respiratory pathogens in clinical care.[1,7] Importantly, patients are commonly infectious and can efficiently transmit the virus during the incubation period before symptom onset.[1,7] This fact is important to remember when considering dynamics of disease spread and from an infection control perspective.

Most patients seem to have a self-limited infection that lasts approximately 3 to 8 days. However, and importantly, patients in certain high-risk categories (including pregnant women) are more likely to suffer from severe complications. Influenza is and should be primarily considered a febrile respiratory illness, with some of those infected showing signs of significant gastrointestinal symptomatology.[1]

The most severe common complication of influenza infection is pneumonia, either primary viral or superimposed bacterial. Viral and bacterial pneumonias can be particularly aggressive, especially during pregnancy and the early postpartum period.[15] Nonrespiratory complications occasionally noted among patients with influenza include pericarditis, myositis, encephalitis, and Guillain-Barre syndrome.

The radiographic findings in primary viral influenza pneumonia are often less extensive than the degree of clinically apparent respiratory compromise. Classically, viral pneumonia is characterized radiographically by diffuse, bilateral, patchy interstitial infiltrates in contrast to the characteristic focal/unilateral infiltrate of bacterial pneumonia. Respiratory failure and acute respiratory distress syndrome (ARDS) can develop. The development of ARDS is thought to be caused by, at least in part, the immune system's overwhelming response to infection. This phenomenon seems to be especially noted during the occasional influenza pandemic.[7,13] When ARDS develops, intensive care support becomes a necessary and life-saving intervention in this small important group of patients. Unfortunately, such patients have a disproportionate contribution from pregnant and early postpartum women.[8,10–14]

Diagnosis of influenza can encompass tests that are available to increase the accuracy of a clinical diagnosis alone. Characteristic symptoms in susceptible patients combined with compatible histories (along with consideration of the seasonal timing) can be reasonably predictive. Rapid influenza tests are available and are often used because they are typically less invasive (nasal/nares swab vs nasopharyngeal swab) and have a short turnaround time. These tests, however, have a low reported sensitivity (40%–60%) despite their high specificity (75%–85%). This combination limits their clinical utility when used as screening tools to rule out infection; these tests can be clinically misleading and should therefore not be relied on to manage high-risk patients.[16] Highly sensitive and specific nasopharyngeal swabs using nucleic acid amplification tests have become the standard test for influenza diagnosis in many locations. Less-invasive, widely available, highly sensitive, and specific tests would be a significant improvement in the care of patients presenting with suggestive clinical syndromes.

IMPACT OF INFLUENZA DURING PREGNANCY

It is clear that pregnant women suffer from disproportionate morbidity, hospitalization rates, and mortality during seasonal outbreaks of influenza and during the occasional influenza pandemic.[8,10–14,17,18] Over the last 5 years (starting with the 2009 H1N1 influenza pandemic), this high-risk status unfortunately has become even clearer in the literature and in clinical settings.[19–22] In addition to the previously documented adverse outcomes among pregnant women, data have emerged showing the impact of influenza in terms of fetal and neonatal effects. These concepts will be further delineated in a later discussion.

Two publications from the influenza pandemic of 1918, or Spanish flu, are the most demonstrative series of the increased risks to pregnant women (both morbidity and mortality) during influenza pandemics. Harris[12] reported on a case series of greater than 1300 pregnant women in the mid-Atlantic region of the United States and documented a 50% mortality rate among pregnant women with Spanish influenza pneumonia. Similarly, Woolston[14] reported the largest single site case series of 101 pregnant women with presumed influenza pneumonia during this same period. Similar to what Harris[12] noted, this cohort also documented an approximate 50% mortality rate among pregnant women compared with the background mortality of approximately 30%. In addition, both investigations documented significantly higher rates of pregnancy complications, such as miscarriage and preterm birth, compared with previous background rates. This phenomenon was especially prominent among women in the third trimester of pregnancy when they contracted pneumonia.[14]

The subsequent influenza pandemic, called the "Asian flu," adds additional historical influenza pandemic data in pregnancy from the 1957 to 1958 season. Greenberg and colleagues[11] noted a highly disproportionate percentage of deaths among pregnant women in New York and an overall increase in maternal mortality (2–3 fold) during the 1957 pandemic. Similarly, Freeman and Barno[10] noted that 50% of the age-grouped deaths in Minnesota came among pregnant women, which typically only comprise 1% of the general population. Influenza pneumonia was associated in both of these investigations with rapid clinical deterioration among pregnant women. When one considers cumulative data from both 20th century pandemics, it is clear that pregnancy increases the risk of morbidity and mortality from influenza and that influenza also imparts negative effects on pregnancy outcomes.

Data from the recent 2009 H1N1 influenza pandemic further bolster these earlier 20th century reports and have increasingly shown adverse pregnancy outcomes from influenza. Within months of the identification of 2009 H1N1, Jamieson and colleagues[13] found that pregnancy again was associated with a heightened risk of hospitalization, severe illness, and mortality. In addition to that publication, numerous additional investigations from many geographic locations showed similar findings and have extended the heightened risks into the early puerperium.

Siston and colleagues[22] reported on more than 750 pregnant women domestically with H1N1 and noted that 5% died, which is at least 5-fold higher than the background rate among the entire population. In addition, as noted above, pregnant women comprise approximately 1% of the population and are thus overrepresented in mortality rates. A separate investigation found that the hospitalization rate was approximately 7 times higher among pregnant women with 2009 H1N1.[19] Louie and colleagues[21] published additional data that importantly highlights that these increases noted in pregnancy seem to extend into the early postpartum period (2 weeks). Additional data originating in Australia show that many of the pregnant women requiring intensive care resources during the 2009 H1N1 pandemic lacked other traditional comorbidities, suggesting pregnancy is the primary driving factor.[20]

Published data and increasingly apparent clinical observation suggest that a portion of the pregnant population seems especially predisposed to rapid clinical deterioration. Frequently, such women present with typical respiratory complaints only to then suffer from rapid decompensation requiring intense support via mechanical ventilation and the use of vasoactive agents, given the frequent septic clinical picture. It is not clear what may predispose such women to the rapid clinical deterioration. Rare clinical and animal data suggest aggressive influenza strains may be noted to have systemic dissemination.[23,24] These data notwithstanding, the contribution of viral systemic dissemination to the pathophysiology of influenza among critically ill pregnant women would benefit from additional study. Furthermore, the precise mechanism(s) placing certain pregnant women at increased risks are not well understood. Pregnancy itself can predispose to worse outcomes for many other viral and bacterial pathogens (eg, varicella, hepatitis E, *Listeria monocytogenes*). Recent attention highlights the potential for specific immunoglobulin G subclass variation to be contributory.[25] Pregnancy is also characterized by changes in immune system function and tolerance as well as marked changes in physiology and altered anatomic considerations of many organ systems that impact respiratory physiology and mechanics.[26,27] Although a precise explanation is currently unclear, it is thought that a combination of pregnancy-specific immune and anatomic/physiologic alterations are what underlie the noted increased susceptibility to worse outcomes from many pathogens in pregnancy.

Reports of seasonal influenza infection during pregnancy also highlight increased risks of cardiopulmonary complications necessitating hospitalization and resource use and higher morbidity during influenza season. Although reports showing higher influenza-attributable morbidity for pregnant women from seasonal epidemics exist, scant data suggest that seasonal epidemics produce disproportionately higher mortality rates in pregnant women.[8,17,18] It is unclear if this finding is caused by lower overall rates of women contracting seasonal infection or less-pathogenic strains. Nevertheless, pregnant women late in gestation with underlying cardiopulmonary conditions seem to be at a particularly increased risk for morbidity and hospitalization. It is the combined pandemic and seasonal data that have produced the long-standing recommendation that pregnant women are a high priority group for receipt of influenza vaccine.[8]

Pneumonia in pregnancy from either bacterial or viral etiology can predispose to preterm birth.[15] Previous data from 20th century pandemics suggested more specifically a fetal/perinatal impact from maternal influenza infection (increased rates of preterm birth and miscarriage). Recent data have focused increasing attention to heightened rates of preterm birth but have also suggested a potential link between maternal influenza infection and fetal growth disturbances.[20,28–30] Multiple investigations have found higher rates of small-for-gestational-age infants born to mothers infected with influenza.[29,30] Additionally, it has also been found that receipt of maternal influenza immunization can lessen the risk of preterm birth by approximately 40%, and small-for-gestational-age status by 30% to 60%.[31,32] Intriguingly, previous epidemiologic data have suggested that maternal influenza infection may predispose to long-term neurologic sequelae among the in utero–exposed fetuses.[33] More recently, a case-control study using banked maternal blood specimens suggested that in utero exposure to maternal influenza may increase one's risk of adult paranoid schizophrenia.[34] Delineation of potential mechanisms for any and all such associations to explain the findings of adverse effects on fetal growth and in utero well-being are not available. These intriguing new findings will undoubtedly continue to be a focus of increasing attention given the focus on optimizing global maternal and neonatal/fetal health.

INFLUENZA PREVENTION

Three basic ways of accomplishing influenza prevention are infection control measures, immunization, and chemoprophylaxis. The latter 2 are discussed here.

Since the 1950s, because of the realization of the increased risks to pregnant women from influenza, inactivated influenza vaccine has been recommended to pregnant women. It remains the most effective manner to prevent disease or minimize the severity of infection. Despite the fact that influenza vaccine has not been specifically studied in pregnancy as part of the US Food and Drug Administration approval process of the various formulations, the greater than 60 years of experience with use of inactivated influenza vaccine in pregnancy has produced a significant body of reassuring safety data.[8,35–39] The overwhelming preponderance of data suggests a very high level of safety for use of the inactivated vaccine in pregnancy, and this information should be shared with all pregnant women. Importantly, the vaccine generates the same robust immune response in pregnant women as it does in nonpregnant women and provides the same level of protection against influenza.[40–42] It is important to re-emphasize here the new data suggesting additional potential benefits (beyond maternal influenza prevention) of maternal receipt of influenza vaccine: preterm birth prevention and a positive impact on fetal growth.[31,32] Clinicians should also understand that the live-attenuated influenza vaccine (FluMist) is not indicated for use in pregnancy, given theoretic concerns about the potential for viremia after immunization. However, if given inadvertently, live-attenuated influenza vaccine does not seem to be harmful and certainly should not prompt pregnancy termination on this basis alone.[43]

Domestic uptake of influenza vaccine in pregnancy has increased over the last few years, undoubtedly fueled by the 2009 H1N1 pandemic and the concomitant focus on pregnant women. For decades, the estimated rates of influenza vaccine uptake in pregnancy hovered at very low percentages, approximately 10% to 20% of the pregnant population.[8,35,44] Starting in 2009, the percentages of pregnant or post-partum women receiving influenza vaccine have increased to approximately 50% and have been maintained around that same level each year since.[45,46] This is clearly progress and is likely multifactorial in origin. However, to sustain and improve these percentages, concerted efforts are required. Reaching the Healthy People 2020 goal of 80% will require continued vigilance on the part of obstetric providers.[47]

The literature on this topic strongly suggests that obstetric providers play a tremendously important role in vaccine uptake by pregnant women. This has been seen in multiple investigations, and it is clear that when obstetric providers recommend and provide the influenza vaccine in their office, the odds of receipt are anywhere from 2 to 50 times higher.[44] Recommendations from obstetric providers about the importance of influenza vaccine during pregnancy should be clear and consistent. Importantly, providers should also include messages about the combined maternal, fetal, and neonatal benefit from maternal immunization.[8,31,32,35,44,48]

Multiple investigations have found that maternal immunization with influenza vaccine also offers neonatal influenza infection prevention. This finding was first noted decades ago in small retrospective analyses that suggested babies born to women who received influenza vaccine in pregnancy had either less severe or delayed onset of influenzalike illnesses.[49,50] In 2008 Zaman and colleagues[48] published results of a prospective, blinded, randomized trial of 340 pregnant women in Bangladesh that showed 63% fewer cases of laboratory-confirmed influenza among infants whose mothers had been immunized compared with infants of women in the control group. Numerous recent observational investigations have likewise shown similar neonatal protective benefits from maternal immunization.[51–53] Maternal passive antibody transmission to the fetus/neonate via the transplacental route currently seems to be the best influenza prevention strategy for newborns because of lack of vaccine approval and use in infants younger than 6 months. Thus, maternal influenza immunization offers demonstrated disease prevention benefits for the mother, fetus, and newborn and is a vital intervention during prenatal care for maternal child health. Given its numerous benefits combined with a relatively low cost of use, it is also a highly cost effective intervention and should be routinely recommended to all pregnant women lacking contraindication.[54]

The other method of influenza infection prevention to review is the use of antiviral drugs after exposure to or close contact with another person/patient with influenza. When considering use of antiviral chemoprophylaxis, it is suggested that obstetric providers elicit complete histories about the nature of the exposure to optimize use in those with a clear risk of disease acquisition. The CDC defines "close contact" as "having cared for or lived with a person who has confirmed, probable, or suspected influenza, or having been in a setting where there was a high likelihood of contact with respiratory droplets and/or body fluids of such a person, including having talked face-to-face with a person with suspected or confirmed influenza illness."[55]

Two classes of anti-influenza medications are currently available for use: the newer neuraminidase inhibitor drugs (oseltamivir and zanamivir) and the older adamantane drugs (amantadine and rimantadine). Oseltamivir (Tamiflu) is currently the most commonly used antiviral medication for influenza treatment and prevention. The neuraminidase inhibitor drugs exert their pharmacologic action by acting as a competitive inhibitor of the influenza viral NA enzyme, which acts on sialic acid. Sialic acid is present on the surface receptors of host cells, and blocking this enzyme prevents new infectious viral particles from being released by infected host cells, which limits or prevents further infectious spread. Since 2009, the adamantanes are not recommended for use because of increasing influenza viral resistance.[6] Oseltamivir (and zanamivir) is currently recommended at an oral dose of 75 mg daily (for 7 days) for the prevention of influenza among exposed individuals based on its 70% to 90% efficacy in preventing infection.[6,56] Because pregnant and immediately postpartum women are at increased risks for severe outcomes from influenza, chemoprophylaxis may be an especially important consideration for clinicians managing such patients. Current knowledge surrounding the safety of these medications (both currently category C) supports their use in pregnancy given the well-documented risks to pregnant women and the absence of any apparent risks from indicated use.[6,57,58] It is likely that with continued use of these medications, additional safety and treatment efficacy data will continue to support use and can also provide a more thorough risk/benefit ratio. The earlier the antiviral is started the better, as the current recommendation is to begin treatment within 48 hours of exposure to maximize potential benefits.[6]

TREATMENT OF INFLUENZA

The foundations for treatment of pregnant women include symptomatic relief with fever reduction, antiviral therapy, and supportive therapy for those few patients with severe disease. The immune system commonly mounts a febrile response to invading pathogens, and influenza is no exception. Fever itself can be uncomfortable for patients, is likely a main driver of seeking care, and has also been suggested to correlate in early pregnancy to an increased risk of neural tube defects.[59] Acetaminophen is the first-line drug for fever in pregnancy and is recommended for use at standard adult doses for pregnant women with fever secondary to influenza.[59]

In terms of antiviral therapy of suspected or proven influenza infection, as noted above, the neuraminidase inhibitors (oseltamivir and zanamivir) are currently the recommended therapy for influenza infection in pregnancy. Published experience with zanamivir in pregnant women is notably limited. Currently it is also recommended to use standard adult dose administration for both drugs when chosen for use in pregnant women.[6] Both drugs have demonstrated efficacy in lessening the duration, severity, and chance of hospitalization from influenza infection in both children and adults with influenza.[6,56,60] Additional systematic review data suggest that both drugs may also lessen the chances of severe illness and hospitalization.[61] Further support to use of neuraminidase inhibitors to prevent more severe infection in pregnancy comes from recent observational data from the 2009 H1N1 influenza pandemic. It has been found that severity of illness among pregnant women in New York City and timing of antiviral treatment are correlated. Pregnant patients who started therapy beyond the 48-hour recommended window of treatment after symptom onset were more likely to have severe influenza illness (3% vs as high as 44% having severe illness, comparing less than 48 hours to greater than 5 days treatment onset, respectively, $P = .002$).[19] Similarly a separate larger investigation of 788 pregnant women with 2009 H1N1 in the United States found a significantly elevated relative risk of 6.0 (95% confidence interval, 3.5–10.6) for admission to the intensive care unit for women treated more than 4 days after symptom onset (compared with <48 hours).[22] These and other clinical data emphasize the importance of a low threshold for early treatment of suspected or confirmed influenza in pregnant women. Moreover, given the currently limited ability to predict which pregnant women may be more susceptible to rapid decompensation and the more than 100-year appreciation that severe outcomes are more likely in pregnancy, universal early treatment should be strongly considered by all obstetric providers in all clinical settings.[56]

It is apparent that pregnant women with influenza are more likely to require critical care resources when compared with the background population. Given the challenge of clinically differentiating primary viral influenza pneumonia, bacterial pneumonia, or a combination, many practitioners prescribe antibiotics empirically along with antiviral drugs to cover for both pathogens until more specific diagnostic information becomes available.[15] The standard approach to the management of critically ill pregnant patients is similar to that of the general population. Stabilization of airway, breathing, and circulatory status is no different in pregnancy. Close attention is given to medication choice (safety considerations) and especially to respiratory status and the potential effects the enlarging gravid uterus during the second and third trimesters of gestation. When faced with recalcitrant and persistently critically ill pregnant women in the latter stages of pregnancy many critical-care clinicians will recommend delivery in hopes of improving respiratory status. This approach attempts to balance the risks of preterm delivery versus the potential for maternal improvement subsequent to relief of the gravid uterus on respiratory function. There are no controlled data to address this specific clinical situation, and it is unlikely that such data will be forthcoming. Case-by-case management with collaboration between high-risk obstetricians and critical care specialists is strongly encouraged to optimize patient outcomes in such clinical scenarios.

SUMMARY

Influenza infection during pregnancy carries disproportionate risks to both mother and baby above and beyond the yearly attributable morbidity and mortality in the general population. This finding is especially apparent during the occasional influenza pandemic. The mechanisms responsible for these increased risks are not fully understood but are likely a combination of the altered physiologic and immunologic parameters of pregnancy. Immunization against influenza is strongly recommended for all pregnant women in any trimester because of its safety, cost effectiveness, and efficacy in preventing influenza in both mothers and newborns. A direct and clear recommendation from an obstetric provider plays a key role in maternal vaccine acceptance. Neuraminidase antiviral medications are indicated during pregnancy and the postpartum period for treatment of confirmed or suspected influenza. Additionally, antiviral medications should also be considered for prophylaxis among pregnant and postpartum women with a history of close contact to a person with influenza.

REFERENCES

1. Treanor J. Influenza virus. In: Mandell GL, Bennett JE, Dolin R, editors. Principles and practice of infectious diseases. Philadelphia: Churchill Livingstone; 2000. p. 1823–49.
2. Estimating seasonal influenza-associated deaths in the United States: CDC study confirms variability of flu. Available at: http://www.cdc.gov/flu/about/disease/us_flu-related_deaths.htm. Accessed June 16, 2014.
3. Adams PF, Hendershot GE, and Marano MA. Current estimates from the National Health Interview Survey, 1996. National Center for Health Statistics. Vital Health Stat 10(200). 1999. Available at: http://www.cdc.gov/nchs/data/series/sr_10/sr10_200.pdf.
4. Molinari NA, Ortega-Sanchez IR, Messonnier ML, et al. The annual impact of seasonal influenza in the US: measuring disease burden and costs. Vaccine 2007;25(27):5086–96.
5. Neumann G, Noda T, Kawaoka Y. Emergence and pandemic potential of swine-origin H1N1 influenza virus. Nature 2009;459(7249):931–9.

6. CDC. 2011–2012 influenza antiviral medications: summary for clinicians. Available at: http://www.cdc.gov/flu/professionals/antivirals/summary-clinicians.htm. Accessed June 16, 2014.
7. Clark NM, Lynch JP. Influenza: epidemiology, clinical features, therapy and prevention. Semin Respir Crit Care Med 2011;32(4):373–92.
8. CDC. Prevention and control of influenza with vaccines. Recommendations of the advisory committee on immunization practices (ACIP), 2010. MMWR Morb Mortal Wkly Rep 2010;59(No. RR-8):1–62.
9. Irving WL, James DK, Stephenson T, et al. Influenza virus infection in the second and third trimesters of pregnancy: a clinical and seroepidemiological study. BJOG 2000;107(10):1282–9.
10. Freeman DW, Barno A. Deaths from Asian influenza associated with pregnancy. Am J Obstet Gynecol 1959;78:1172–5.
11. Greenberg M, Jacobziner H, Pakter J, et al. Maternal mortality in the epidemic of Asian influenza, New York City, 1957. Am J Obstet Gynecol 1958;76:897–902.
12. Harris J. Influenza occurring in pregnant women: a statistical study of thirteen hundred and fifty cases. JAMA 1919;72:978–80.
13. Jamieson DJ, Honein MA, Rasmussen SA, et al. H1N1 2009 influenza virus infection during pregnancy in the USA. Lancet 2009;374(9688):451–8.
14. Woolston DC. Epidemic pneumonia (Spanish Influenza) in pregnancy: effect in one hundred and one cases. JAMA 1918;71:1898–9.
15. Sheffield JS, Cunningham FG. Community-acquired pneumonia in pregnancy. Obstet Gynecol 2009;114(4):915–22.
16. CDC. Evaluation of rapid influenza diagnostic tests for detection of novel influenza A (H1N1) virus – United States, 2009. MMWR Morb Mortal Wkly Rep 2009;58(30):826–9.
17. Cox S, Posner SF, Mcpheeters M, et al. Hospitalizations with respiratory illness among pregnant women during influenza season. Obstet Gynecol 2006;107(6): 1315–22.
18. Neuzil KM, Reed GW, Mitchel EF, et al. Impact of influenza on acute cardiopulmonary hospitalizations in pregnant women. Am J Epidemiol 1998;148(11): 1094–102.
19. Creanga AA, Johnson TF, Graitcer SB, et al. Severity of 2009 pandemic influenza A (H1N1) virus infection in pregnant women. Obstet Gynecol 2010; 115(4):717–26.
20. Hewagama S, Walker SP, Stuart RL, et al. 2009 H1N1 influenza A and pregnancy outcomes in Victoria, Australia. Clin Infect Dis 2010;50(5):686–90.
21. Louie JK, Acosta M, Jamieson DJ, et al, California Pandemic Working Group. Severe 2009 H1N1 influenza in pregnant and postpartum women in California. N Engl J Med 2010;362(1):27–35.
22. Siston AM, Rasmussen SA, Honein MA, et al. Pandemic 2009 influenza A(H1N1) virus illness among pregnant women in the United States. JAMA 2010;303(15): 1517–25.
23. Sweet C, Toms FL, Smith H. The pregnant ferret as a model for studying the congenital effects of influenza virus infection in utero: infection of foetal tissues in organ culture and in vivo. Br J Exp Pathol 1977;58:113–23.
24. Shu Y, Yu H, Li D. Lethal avian influenza A (H5N1) infection in a pregnant woman in Anhui Province, China. N Engl J Med 2006;354(3):1421–2.
25. Gordon CL, Johnson PD, Permezel M, et al. Association between severe pandemic 2009 influenza A (H1N1) virus infection and immunoglobulin G(2) subclass deficiency. Clin Infect Dis 2010;50(5):672–8.

26. Anderson GD. Pregnancy-induced changes in pharmacokinetics: a mechanistic-based approach. Clin Pharmacokinet 2005;44(10):989–1008.
27. Weinberg ED. Pregnancy-associated depression of cell-mediated immunity. Rev Infect Dis 1984;6:814–31.
28. Goodnight WH, Soper DE. Pneumonia in Pregnancy. Crit Care Med 2005;33(10 Suppl):S390–7.
29. McNeil SA, Dodds LA, Fell DB, et al. Effect of respiratory hospitalization during pregnancy on infant outcomes. Am J Obstet Gynecol 2011;204(6 Suppl 1): S54–7.
30. Naresh A, Fisher BM, Hoppe KK, et al. A multicenter cohort study of pregnancy outcomes among with laboratory-confirmed 2009 H1N1 infection. J Perinatol 2013;33(12):939–43.
31. Omer SB, Goodman D, Steinhoff MC, et al. Maternal influenza immunization and reduced likelihood of prematurity and small for gestational age births: a retrospective cohort study. PLoS Med 2011;8(5):e1000441.
32. Steinhoff MC, Omer SB, Roy E, et al. Neonatal outcomes after influenza immunization during pregnancy: a randomized controlled trial. CMAJ 2012;184(6): 645–53.
33. Mednick SA, Machon RA, Huttenen MO, et al. Adult schizophrenia following prenatal exposure to an influenza epidemic. Arch Gen Psychiatry 1988;45:189–92.
34. Brown AS, Begg MD, Gravenstein S, et al. Serologic evidence of prenatal influenza in the etiology of schizophrenia. Arch Gen Psychiatry 2004;61:774–80.
35. Mak TK, Mangtani P, Leese J, et al. Influenza vaccination in pregnancy:current evidence and selected national policies. Lancet Infect Dis 2008;8(1):44–52.
36. Tamma PD, Ault KA, del Rio C, et al. Safety of influenza vaccine in pregnancy. Am J Obstet Gynecol 2009;201(6):547–52.
37. Carcione D, Blyth CC, Richmond PC, et al. Safety surveillance of influenza vaccine in pregnant women. Aust N Z J Obstet Gynaecol 2013;53(1):98–9.
38. Bednarczyk RA, Adjaye-Gbewonyo D, Omer SB. Safety of influenza immunization during pregnancy for the fetus and the neonate. Am J Obstet Gynecol 2012; 207(3 Suppl):S38–46.
39. Moro PL, Broder K, Zheteyeva Y, et al. Adverse events in pregnant women following administration of trivalent inactivated influenza vaccine and live attenuated influenza vaccine in the Vaccine Adverse Event Reporting System, 1990–2009. Am J Obstet Gynecol 2011;204:146.e1–7.
40. Englund JA, Mbawuike IN, Hammil H, et al. Maternal immunization with influenza or tetanus toxoid vaccine for passive antibody protection in young infants. J Infect Dis 1993;168(3):647–56.
41. Jackson L, Patel SM, Swamy GK, et al. Immunogenicity of an inactivated monovalent 2009 H1N1 influenza vaccine in pregnant women. J Infect Dis 2011; 204(6):854–63.
42. Thompson MG, Li DK, Shifflett P, et al. Effectiveness of seasonal trivalent influenza vaccine for preventing influenza virus illness among pregnant women: a population-based case-control study during the 2010-2011 and 2011-2012 influenza seasons. Clin Infect Dis 2014;58:449–57.
43. Toback SL, Beigi R, Tennis P, et al. Maternal outcomes among pregnant women receiving live attenuated influenza vaccine. Influenza Other Respir Viruses 2012;6(1):44–51.
44. Shavell VI, Moniz MH, Gonik B, et al. Influenza immunization in pregnancy: overcoming patient and health care provider barriers. Am J Obstet Gynecol 2012; 207(3 Suppl):S67–74.

45. Centers for Disease Control and Prevention (CDC). Pregnant women and flu vaccination, internet panel survey, United States, November 2013a. Available at: http://www.cdc.gov/flu/fluvaxview/pregnant-women-nov2013.htm. Accessed June 25, 2014.

46. Centers for Disease Control and Prevention (CDC). Prevention and control of seasonal influenza with vaccines. Recommendations of the Advisory Committee on Immunization Practices–United States, 2013-2014. MMWR Recomm Rep 2013;62(RR-07):1–43.

47. Healthy people 2020 topics and objectives: immunizations and infectious diseases, IID-12.10. Available at: http://www.healthypeople.gov/2020/topics-objectives2020/objectiveslist.aspx?topicId=23. Accessed June 26, 2014.

48. Zaman K, Roy E, Arifeen SE, et al. Effectiveness of maternal influenza immunization in mothers and infants. N Engl J Med 2008;359:1555–64.

49. Puck JM, Glezen WP, Frank AL, et al. Protection of infants from infection with influenza A virus by transplacentally acquired antibody. J Infect Dis 1980; 142(6):844–9.

50. Reuman PD, Ayoub EM, Small PA. Effect of passive maternal antibody on influenza illness in children: a prospective study of influenza A in mother-infant pairs. Pediatr Infect Dis J 1987;6(4):398–403.

51. Eick AA, Uyeki TM, Klimov A, et al. Maternal influenza vaccination and effect on influenza virus infection in young infants. Arch Pediatr Adolesc Med 2011;165: 104–11.

52. Benowitz I, Esposito DB, Gracey KD, et al. Influenza vaccine given to pregnant women reduces hospitalization due to influenza in their infants. Clin Infect Dis 2010;51:1355–61.

53. Poehling KA, Szilagyi PG, Staat MA, et al. Impact of maternal immunization on influenza hospitalizations in infants. Am J Obstet Gynecol 2011;204(6 Suppl 1):S141–8.

54. Beigi R, Wiringa AE, Bailey RR, et al. Economic value of seasonal an pandemic influenza vaccination among pregnant women. Clin Infect Dis 2009;49(12):1784–92.

55. CDC. Updated recommendations for obstetric health care providers related to use of antiviral medications in the treatment and prevention of influenza for the 2013-2014 season. Available at: http://www.cdc.gov/flu/professionals/antivirals/avrec_ob2011.htm. Accessed July 7, 2014.

56. Jefferson T, Demicheli V, Deeks J, et al. Neuraminidase inhibitors for preventing and treating influenza in healthy adults. Cochrane Database Syst Rev 2000;(2):CD001265.

57. Tanaka T, Nakajima K, Murashima A, et al. Safety of neuraminidase inhibitors against novel influenza A (H1N1) in pregnant and breastfeeding women. CMAJ 2009;181(1–2):55–8.

58. Greer LG, Sheffield JS, Rogers VL, et al. Maternal and neonatal outcomes after antepartum treatment of influenza with antiviral medications. Obstet Gynecol 2010;115:711–6.

59. Rasmussen SA, Jamieson DJ, Macfarlane K, et al. Pandemic influenza and pregnant women: summary of a meeting of experts. Am J Public Health 2009; 99(Suppl 2):S248–54.

60. Matheson NJ, Symmonds-Abrahams M, Sheikh A, et al. Neuraminidase inhibitors for preventing and treating influenza in children. Cochrane Database Syst Rev 2003;(3):CD002744.

61. Hsu J, Santesso N, Mustafa R, et al. Antivirals for treatment of influenza: a systematic review and meta-analysis of observational studies. Ann Intern Med 2012;156(7):512–24.

Contemporary Management of Human Immunodeficiency Virus in Pregnancy

 CrossMark

Meghan Donnelly, MD[a], Jill K. Davies, MD[b],*

KEYWORDS

- HIV • Pregnancy • Perinatal transmission • Vertical transmission
- Mother to child transmission • Perinatal infection

KEY POINTS

- Although new infections in women seem to be decreasing in the United States, a significant number of infected individuals are estimated to be unaware of their status. Universal opt-out HIV testing in pregnancy, including rapid testing intrapartum, identifies the most number of gravidas with HIV infection. HIV testing of high-risk women should be repeated in the third trimester.

- Preconception counseling for HIV-infected women is critical, and reproductive-aged men and women living with HIV should have conversations about their reproductive desires at every visit, with appropriate methods of contraception advised until conditions for pregnancy are optimized.

- All pregnant women should be offered combined antiretroviral therapy (cART) during pregnancy regardless of HIV disease status to maximize maternal health and decrease perinatal transmission.

- Women with viral loads greater than or equal to 1000 copies/mL should be offered cesarean delivery at 38 weeks to decrease the risk of perinatal transmission associated with vaginal delivery. Invasive monitoring techniques, such as intrauterine pressure catheter or fetal scalp electrode use, and operative vaginal delivery should be avoided because they can increase risk of perinatal transmission.

Continued

Disclosures/Conflict of Interest: The authors have no disclosures or conflicts of interests to report.
[a] Department of Obstetrics and Gynecology, University of Colorado Health, University of Colorado Denver School of Medicine, 12631 East 17th Avenue, Aurora, CO 80045, USA;
[b] Department of Obstetrics & Gynecology, Denver Health Medical Center, University of Colorado Denver School of Medicine, 12631 East 17th Avenue, Aurora, CO 80045, USA
* Corresponding author. Denver Health Medical Center, 777 Bannock Street, MC 0660, Denver, CO 80204.
E-mail address: Jill.davies@dhha.org

Obstet Gynecol Clin N Am 41 (2014) 547–571
http://dx.doi.org/10.1016/j.ogc.2014.08.003
0889-8545/14/$ – see front matter © 2014 Elsevier Inc. All rights reserved.

obgyn.theclinics.com

Continued

- Providers should have a frank, culturally sensitive discussion with their patients regarding breastfeeding. Although breastfeeding is universally discouraged in settings where formula feeding is safe, women experience significant guilt about not breastfeeding. Thus, psychosocial support may help to prevent unintended perinatal transmission through breastfeeding.
- All methods of contraception are available to human immunodeficiency virus (HIV)-infected women. Some ARV regimens may influence the metabolism of hormonal contraception and dosing modification may be suggested. For prevention of transmission to sexual partners, regular and consistent condom use should be advised.

INTRODUCTION

Human immunodeficiency infection was first described in 1981, and in 1983 a novel retrovirus, named *human immunodeficiency virus*, was identified as the infectious agent. This disease was initially documented in risk groups, including men who have sex with men, intravenous (IV) drug users, and hemophiliacs, but then was also reported in women and infants.[1] Now, more than 3 decades later, perinatal transmission in resource-rich settings has become uncommon and the goal of elimination of perinatal HIV transmission may be possible in the foreseeable future.[2–4]

This review covers key concepts in the pathophysiology of HIV, with emphasis on perinatal transmission, and reviews appropriate screening and diagnostic testing for HIV during pregnancy. Current recommendations for medical, pharmacologic, and obstetric management of women newly diagnosed with HIV during pregnancy and women with preexisting infection, with an emphasis on the resource-rich setting, are also discussed. Preconception counseling for HIV-positive women and postpartum issues are addressed.

Compared with an early incidence of perinatal transmission of HIV as high as 42%, the introduction of antepartum and intrapartum ARV therapy and postnatal prophylaxis of infants has led to near eradication of perinatal transmission, recognized as one of the greatest medical achievements thus far in the twenty-first century.[5]

DISEASE DESCRIPTION (HUMAN IMMUNODEFICIENCY VIRUS AND AIDS)

From the family of retroviruses, HIV-1 and less commonly HIV-2 cause acquired immunodeficiency. Replication of the virus and integration into the host genome cause progressive depletion of CD4 cells, leading clinically to increased risk for opportunistic infections and AIDS. A detailed description of this disease is outside the scope of this article.

HIV has been isolated from many human bodily fluids, including blood, seminal fluid, pre-ejaculate, cerebrospinal fluid, saliva, tears, and breast milk. Additionally, HIV is found in both cell-free and cell-associated fractions.[1,6]

The Centers for Disease Control and Prevention (CDC) recently revised the case definition of HIV and stage of disease classification, such that the disease is classified into 5 infection stages, graded 0 to 3 plus unknown. The higher the number, the more advanced the disease based on CD4$^+$ count. Opportunistic infections occur during stage 3. This classification is primarily used for public health surveillance and is less relevant to clinical care.[7]

RISK FACTORS

Sexual transmission is currently the most prevalent method of spread of HIV infection, both globally and in the United States. Sexual transmission of HIV has been associated with certain sexual behaviors, such as penile-anal intercourse and penile-vaginal intercourse, more commonly than oral sex. Risk factors for nonsexual transmission include infection with contaminated blood products; injection drug use; occupational exposures, such as accidental needle sticks; and perinatal transmission.[6] Additionally, many individuals who acquired HIV through perinatal transmission are now of reproductive age themselves. Because of their number of years of infection, these patients represent a particularly challenging subset to treat.

Other risk factors facilitating transmission can be categorized into infectiousness of the host, susceptibility of the recipient, and viral properties. A host is more infectious, with more advanced stage of infection as measured by $CD4^+$ count or high viral load as well as exposure during primary infection. Factors that improve $CD4^+$ count and diminish viral load substantially decrease this risk. Susceptibility of the recipient is associated with risk factors for sexual transmission, such as genital ulcer disease and other sexually transmitted infections, as well as trauma during sexual contact.

Proper and consistent barrier methods of contraception mitigate risk for sexual transmission. Among serodiscordant couples, recent studies have demonstrated that earlier initiation of ARV therapy (ART) in an infected partner ($CD4^+$ counts of 350–550 cells/mm^3) and pre-exposure prophylaxis of an uninfected partner reduce risk for sexual acquisition of HIV. Although effective methods of contraception, hormonal contraception, such as oral contraceptives and depot medroxyprogesterone acetate, may increase the risk for HIV acquisition.[8]

Pregnancy has also been suggested as a time of increased susceptibility for HIV acquisition, attributed to alterations in the immune system and endocrinologic changes. Pregnancy also represents a time when condom use may be less common in at-risk individuals. Thus, provider surveillance of high-risk women during pregnancy and postpartum during breastfeeding is critical for prevention of seroconversion during this high-risk time. Provider recognition of symptoms consistent with primary HIV infection and similar education of at-risk patients alert both provider and patient when primary infection may have occurred so that appropriate testing can be performed. Risk factors for perinatal transmission of HIV are discussed later.

EPIDEMIOLOGY

Approximately 75 million people worldwide have been infected with HIV since the epidemic began and 36 million have succumbed to AIDS-related deaths. In 2012, 35.3 million individuals are estimated to be living with HIV. Encouragingly, the number of new infections overall has decreased by 33% since 2001 and the number of new infections in children has diminished by 52% in the same time period. Additionally, a 29% decrease in AIDS-related deaths has been noted in adults and children since 2005. This is likely related to the 40-fold increase in access to ARV therapy between 2002 and 2012, including tremendous reductions in cost per person. In 2012, 62% of pregnant women living in epidemic countries were estimated to have access to these medications, with many countries reporting upwards of 80% who have access to ARV treatment. On the other hand, it is estimated that as many as 50% of people living with HIV globally are unaware of their status.[9]

In the United States, the CDC estimates that 1.1 million are living with HIV based on 2011 reporting (**Fig. 1**). Alarmingly, it is suggested that 1 in 6 is unaware of their infection. Infections among women are stabilizing in the United States after approximately a

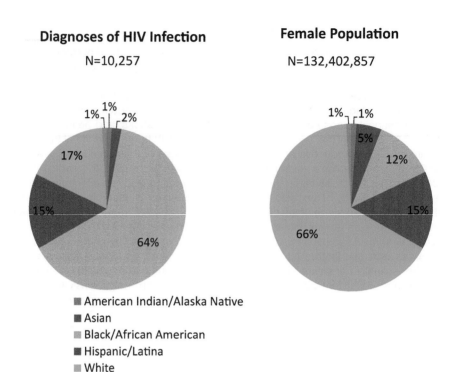

Diagnoses of HIV Infection
N=10,257

Female Population
N=132,402,857

■ American Indian/Alaska Native
■ Asian
■ Black/African American
■ Hispanic/Latina
■ White
■ Multiple Races

Fig. 1. Diagnosis of HIV infection and population among female adults and adolescents, by race/ethnicity, 2011—United States. (*From* National Center for HIV/AIDS, Viral Hepatitis, STD & TB Prevention, Division of HIV/AIDS Prevention. Centers for Disease Control. HIV surveillance by race/ethnicity. Available at: http://www.cdc.gov/hiv/pdf/statistics_surveillance_raceethnicity.pdf. Accessed August 13, 2014.)

decade of increasing prevalence, with women representing 24% of all HIV infections in 2009. However, 9500 new infections were reported in women in 2010 and this represents a 21% decline over the 12,000 new infections reported in 2009. Overall, women represent 20% of new infections in 2010. Heterosexual contact is the contributory cause in 84% of these, with the remaining 16% attributed to IV drug use.[10]

Latinos and black women remain over-represented in those living with HIV. In 2011, female black/African Americans made up 12% of the female population in the United States but accounted for an estimated 64% of diagnoses of HIV infection among girls and women. Female Hispanics/Latinos made up 15% of the female population in the United States and accounted for 15% of diagnoses of HIV infection among girls and women. White females made up 66% of the female adult and adolescent population in the United States but accounted only for 17% of diagnoses of HIV infection among girls and women.[11]

Data on perinatal transmission from 2008 to 2010 report a 16% reduction in perinatally acquired HIV infections (www.cdc.gov/hiv/pdf/policies_NationalProgressReport. Centers for Disease Control and Prevention. *National HIV Prevention Progress Report, 2013*). In 2010, there were 212 cases of perinatal transmission in the United States, again with black/African Americans overrepresented.[12] These infections are considered missed opportunities and may even be considered sentinel events.

PATHOGENESIS OF PERINATAL TRANSMISSION OF HUMAN IMMUNODEFICIENCY VIRUS

Perinatal transmission of HIV is hypothesized to occur

1. During pregnancy by direct hematogenous, transplacental spread or ascending infection from virus in the genital tract into amniotic fluid and membranes
2. Intrapartum
    a. Through mucocutaneous contact of the fetus with maternal blood, amniotic fluid, and genital tract secretions
    b. Through ascending infection from the cervicovaginal secretions
    c. From uterine contractions leading to maternal fetal microtransfusions of blood
3. To infants via breastfeeding

In nonbreastfeeding populations, approximately one-third of transmission is attributed to in utero infection whereas the remaining two-thirds is estimated to occur intrapartum. Data to support these approximations come from timing of seroconversion in the newborn and infant periods in the first 2 days of life versus after the first week of life. Other investigators have suggested, however, that up to one-half of perinatal transmission occurs in late pregnancy prior to the onset of labor. It is also suggested that HIV virus in either cell-free fractions or cell-associated virus may be present in the fetal circulation but not integrated into the host. Although biologically active, if the fetal immune system is not activated, the virus decays over time and may not establish infection until a later time, if at all. It may be the labor process that causes fetal immune system activation and integration of the virus into the host genome.[13]

Factors influencing perinatal HIV transmission include[13]

Viral factors
- Viral load in plasma, genitourinary tract, and breast milk
- Viral characteristics: genotype, phenotype, tropism, resistance to ARV agents, and capacity for immune escape

Host factors

Immunologic factors
- Maternal CD4 count/stage of HIV disease
- Maternal immune factors (such as neutralizing antibodies)
- Breast milk immune factors
- Fetal/neonatal immune response (such as cytotoxic lymphocyte response)

Genetic factors
- Fetal HLA type, maternal-fetal HLA concordance, and single nucleotide polymorphisms for chemokines/chemokine receptors/innate immune factors

Tissue/mucosal integrity
- Chorioamnionitis/placental pathology/maturational stage
- Maternal genitourinary lesions/sexually transmitted diseases
- Cracked or bleeding nipples/breast abscess/clinical or subclinical mastitis
- Barrier integrity (neonatal skin and mucosal membranes)
- Infant gastrointestinal maturity
- Vitamin A/other micronutrient deficiency

Obstetric factors
- Mode of delivery
- Timing of delivery
- Invasive monitoring/obstetric procedures
- Duration of membrane rupture

Acute HIV infection during pregnancy is associated with a higher risk for perinatal transmission, because it is associated with a much higher viral load. Obstetric care providers should be familiar with signs and symptoms of primary infection and have a high level of suspicion for repeat HIV testing during pregnancy or breastfeeding in such situations, particularly those with high-risk factors. Those risk factors would include those who are incarcerated or who receive care at facilities with an incidence of greater than or equal to 1/1000 pregnant women, or those acquiring other sexually transmitted infections during pregnancy. Approximately 40% to 90% of patients experiencing acute HIV infection experience symptoms, such as fever, lymphadenopathy, pharyngitis, skin rash, and myalgias/arthralgias, among others. When HIV antigen/antibody tests results are negative or indeterminate in this setting, HIV RNA viral load testing should be performed and viral load in this setting is generally high, greater than 100,000 copies/mL.[14] A recent abstract presentation suggested that perinatal transmission of HIV is 8-fold higher in women who seroconverted during pregnancy.[15]

PRECONCEPTION COUNSELING, EFFECTS OF PREGNANCY ON HUMAN IMMUNODEFICIENCY VIRUS AND HUMAN IMMUNODEFICIENCY VIRUS EFFECTS ON PREGNANCY

Increasing fertility desires in those living with HIV has been addressed in recent literature.[16] Additionally, a US study demonstrated that 83% of pregnancies in HIV-infected pregnant adolescents were unplanned,[17] as were 58% of pregnancies in an Italian study of HIV-infected women on ART.[18] A discussion tool for patients and primary HIV care providers is described in A Guide to the Clinical Care of Women with HIV/AIDS (available through the Web site, www.hab.hrsa.gov).[8] For women not currently interested in becoming pregnant, this tool usually is sufficient for assessment. For those women with desire to conceive in the near future, those on ART agents with teratogenic potential, those in serodiscordant relationships, or those with significant medical problems, however, referral to obstetrics/gynecology or maternal-fetal medicine is recommended.

An outline for comprehensive preconception evaluation is reproduced as Appendix A, from A Guide to the Clinical Care of Women with HIV/AIDS.[8] Optimization of a woman's HIV disease, modification of ART regimen, and improving comorbid medical conditions and appropriate contraception until conception is safer can be facilitated during a preconception visit (discussed later). Sexually transmitted infections can be screened for and treated. Immunizations can be facilitated at that visit as well as interventions, such as smoking cessation, screening for alcohol/substance use/abuse, assessment and treatment of mental illness, and providing prescriptions for prenatal vitamins containing at least 400 μg/d of folic acid.

For those in serodiscordant couples desiring to conceive, expert consultation is recommended to further outline options available to minimize both horizontal and perinatal transmission. A detailed discussion of options from timed unprotected intercourse during the ovulatory window to advanced reproductive techniques as well as pre-exposure prophylaxis should be addressed in such a consultation and an individualized plan suggested. Further detail on these options is beyond the scope of this review, but readers are referred to a recent review on this topic by Savasi and colleagues.[19] Given the increased risk for infertility in both HIV-infected men and women, centers with specific expertise in this area should be sought. Perinatal HIV/AIDS Clinician Consultation Center at the University of California, San Francisco (1-888-448-8765 and at nccc.ucsf. edu), maintains a list of centers providing these services.

A discussion of the effects of pregnancy on HIV infection and the effects of HIV infection on pregnancy is critical to the preconception counseling visit for women living with HIV. A decline in absolute CD4 count is often seen, attributed to volume expansion in pregnancy with concomitant hemodilution; the CD4$^+$ percentage remains stable so may be a better marker to follow in pregnancy. If not on ARV therapy, HIV viral load remains stable during pregnancy but may increase transiently postpartum. The clinical course of infection is not thought adversely affected by pregnancy compared with women who do not experience pregnancy.[8]

Also relevant to this discussion is whether HIV changes the risk for adverse pregnancy outcomes outside perinatal transmission risk. Most of the literature suggests that HIV-related confounders, such as advanced disease, anemia, and malnutrition, may increase the risk of prematurity and thus perinatal morbidity and mortality. Similarly, the literature also supports that after controlling for social factors, such as tobacco, alcohol, illicit drug use, and scant prenatal care, HIV does not independently increase adverse pregnancy outcomes.[8,20]

For serodiscordant couples, it is important to emphasize continued consistent condom use during pregnancy because this may be a time where couples are less likely to use them, and male-to-female transmissions have occurred. More recently, an increased risk of female-to-male transmission during pregnancy has been suggested.[21]

Until a woman with HIV meets criteria to become pregnant, it is her care provider's responsibility to assure appropriate contraception and address this at each visit.

Effects of Human Immunodeficiency Virus and Pregnancy on Other Infections

Because both pregnancy and HIV infection are associated with increased symptomatic *Candida* infections, pregnant women with HIV infection should be symptomatically screened and treated for vulvovaginal candidiasis. Because of potential systemic interactions with ART, topical agents are preferentially recommended for treatment. With potential for persistent infections, topical therapy for at least 7 days is recommended. Prophylaxis should be considered when systemic antibiotics are prescribed.[8] Bacterial vaginosis (BV) has been associated with an increased risk for perinatal HIV transmission and increased prevalence in HIV-infected women. BV may be more difficult to eradicate in HIV-infected women. Pregnant women living with HIV should be asked about signs and symptoms of vaginal infections with screening performed in symptomatic women with treatment when BV is identified. Systemic treatment with oral metronidazole or clindamycin is recommended.[8]

Because of common coinfection with genital herpes,[22] as well as more frequent, severe, and protracted episodes in HIV-infected women and reactivation in labor, screening for type-specific herpes simplex virus (HSV) antibodies may be helpful to guide pregnancy management, especially if a partner is known to be HSV positive.[22] Because of the association of HSV with increased risk for perinatal HIV transmission prior to cART,[23] and the association between HSV prophylaxis to reduce viral shedding and symptomatic infections at the time of labor, offering HSV prophylaxis in the late third trimester seems low risk and of significant potential benefit.[23] It is unclear if late third-trimester HSV prophylaxis will further reduce the already low risk of perinatal HIV transmission with cART. Following American College of Obstetricians and Gynecologists (ACOG) guidelines regarding mode of delivery and active lesions is recommended.[8,24]

Due to the immunodeficiency associated with HIV infection, screening for cytomegalovirus (CMV) and toxoplasmosis during pregnancy in HIV-infected women is recommended. Additionally, precautions to prevent CMV and toxoplasmosis acquisition during pregnancy seem prudent.

The seroprevalence of hepatitis C is estimated at 17% to 54% in HIV-infected pregnant women.[25] HIV is thought to increase perinatal transmission of hepatitis C to 10% to

20%.[26,27] Coinfection is also suspected to increase HIV perinatal transmission. Hepatitis C coinfection should not, however, influence mode of delivery recommendations. Pregnancy management of hepatitis C is unaltered. Although there are numerous newer antivirals now available for hepatitis C, the experience with their use in pregnancy is unknown and is not currently recommended.[8] Given the complex issues in hepatitis coinfections with HIV, expert consultation is recommended to help manage these patients.

There seems to be no difference in group B streptococcus (GBS) colonization rates between HIV-1–positive and HIV-1–negative pregnant women.[28] Standard screening and prophylaxis for GBS in pregnancy applies.

DIAGNOSIS/TESTING

There are 2 strategies for HIV testing in pregnancy: opt-in, in which pregnant women are given pre-HIV test counseling and then must agree to receiving the test, and opt-out, in which women are informed that HIV testing is included in the standard prenatal laboratory panel given to all pregnant women with the option to decline HIV testing if they so desire. At the Denver Health Medical Center, 98.2% of women who delivered between 1998 and 2001 received HIV testing using opt out testing.[29] The CDC recommends, and many states now mandate, opt-out testing for all pregnant women in early pregnancy, as well as retesting in the third trimester for women who live in geographic areas of high HIV prevalence or are otherwise considered at high risk for HIV exposure. Rapid HIV screening of who present to labor and delivery without a previous test performed or ongoing risk without repeat testing is recommended.[30] Further information for HIV testing laws during pregnancy in each state can be found at http://nccc.ucsf.edu/clinical-resources/hiv-aids-resources/state-hiv-testing-laws.

In addition to performing opt-out testing, it is important to examine and address the reasons why women decline testing. Common provider-related barriers are language differences, late or no prenatal care, low perception of patient risk, or the recommendation for testing is not universally offered. Patient barriers include perception that they are not at risk, poor understanding of risk of HIV to patients and infants, or fear of negative consequences of testing, such as social stigmatization and damage to relationships. Studies have shown that strong provider recommendation is associated with higher rates of testing.[31,32]

Draft recommendations from the CDC in 2012[33] advocate using a fourth-generation immunoassay to screen for acute HIV-1 infections and established HIV-1 and HIV-2 infections (Fig. 2).[33] The fourth-generation test differs from previous-generation tests in that it contains synthetic peptide or recombinant protein antigens as well as p24 antibody and thus is designed to detect IgM and IgG antibodies and the p24 antigen so that patients test positive more rapidly after seroconversion than with previous-generation assays. If a patient tests positive for HIV with this assay, it is recommended to proceed to an HIV-1/HIV-2 antibody differentiation immunoassay. Patients who test positive for HIV-1 or HIV-2 at this step should then proceed with supplemental laboratory testing, such as viral load and CD4 lymphocyte counts, to stage disease and initiate treatment. Patients who test negative in the antibody differentiation immunoassay should have an RNA viral load (nucleic acid testing) performed. If this is positive, it indicates an acute HIV-1 infection. If negative, there was likely a false-positive result on the initial assay or, rarely in the United States, acute infection with HIV-2.

The Western blot (WB) is left out of this CDC testing algorithm. WBs are prone to indeterminate results due to several factors, including cross-reactivity of nonspecific antibodies (particularly in pregnancy), recent exposure/current seroconversion, infection with HIV-2, or technical error. The fourth-generation screening test maximizes

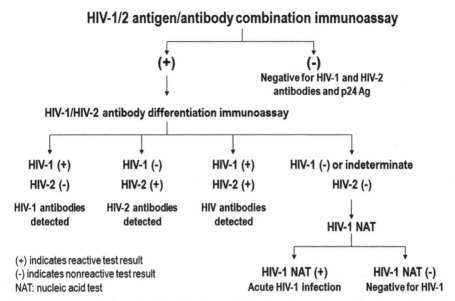

HIV-1/2 antigen/antibody combination immunoassay

(+)

(-) Negative for HIV-1 and HIV-2 antibodies and p24 Ag

HIV-1/HIV-2 antibody differentiation immunoassay

HIV-1 (+) **HIV-2 (-)**
HIV-1 antibodies detected

HIV-1 (-) **HIV-2 (+)**
HIV-2 antibodies detected

HIV-1 (+) **HIV-2 (+)**
HIV antibodies detected

HIV-1 (-) or indeterminate **HIV-2 (-)**
HIV-1 NAT

(+) indicates reactive test result
(-) indicates nonreactive test result
NAT: nucleic acid test

HIV-1 NAT (+) Acute HIV-1 infection

HIV-1 NAT (-) Negative for HIV-1

Fig. 2. Recommended testing algorithm for HIV infection. (*From* Centers for Disease Control and Prevention and Association of Public Health Laboratories. Laboratory Testing for the Diagnosis of HIV Infection: Updated Recommendations. Available at http://stacks.cdc.gov/view/cdc/23447. Published June 27, 2014. Accessed September 30, 2014.)

sensitivity, whereas using a second-generation immunoblot, such as Multispot, identifies HIV-2 infections in addition to HIV-1, is less expensive, and allows more rapid identification of true positives compared with WB. Standard testing algorithms recommend patients should not be notified that they are HIV-positive until confirmatory testing is returned. Rapid HIV testing performed on labor and delivery is an exception to this, because treatment to prevent intrapartum transmission should not be delayed while waiting for confirmatory testing.[33]

INDICATIONS FOR THERAPY

HIV therapy in pregnancy is directed at 2 separate but complementary aims: therapy to optimize maternal health and therapy to prevent perinatal transmission. The overarching goal, however, is to prevent toxic or subtherapeutic treatment of the mother or fetus antepartum, intrapartum, and postpartum to improve outcomes for both patients. Currently, the consensus recommendation is to treat all HIV-infected pregnant women with cART, regardless of their CD4 count or viral load, to prevent perinatal transmission. This guideline differs from those guiding treatment outside of pregnancy because there have been cases of perinatal transmission reported with low or undetectable plasma maternal viral loads[34–36] and there is accumulating evidence that plasma viral load may not be entirely reflective of genital shedding and risk of intrapartum perinatal transmission.[37,38]

GUIDELINES FOR ANTEPARTUM ANTIRETROVIRAL THERAPY/PREGNANCY CONSIDERATIONS

In general, the same treatment considerations used to guide therapy for HIV infection outside of pregnancy should be applied to pregnant women. Changes in maternal physiology during pregnancy, however, lead to pharmacokinetic changes that may result in subtherapeutic drug levels and to fetal concerns and perinatal transmission risk that must be taken into account. As new ARV medications are rapidly expanding pharmacologic treatment options, there are often few pregnancy data available for these newer agents. Perinatal HIV/AIDS Clinician Consultation Center provides clinical consultation antepartum, intrapartum, or for the neonate, free of charge. Additionally, the Antiretroviral Pregnancy Registry is another useful resource for accessing information about the effects of ARV drugs in pregnancy. The registry allows providers to enroll their patients to prospectively collect as much data as possible to detect teratogenicity or adverse pregnancy outcome caused by ARV drugs as early as possible. This registry can be accessed at www.APRegistry.com.[39]

Perinatal transmission can occur during pregnancy, during delivery, or postpartum with breastfeeding; thus, treatment strategies to prevent perinatal transmission must take these 3 time periods into consideration. In addition to lowering maternal plasma viral load and genital tract shedding, many ARV drugs cross the placenta to achieve adequate antepartum fetal levels, providing infant pre-exposure prophylaxis[40] as well as postexposure prophylaxis in the newborn.[40]

As early as the first trimester, pregnant women develop increased body water and fat, increased blood volume, increased glomerular filtration, increased cardiac output, and slowed gastrointestinal transit times. Coupling these changes with the significant nausea and vomiting that often occur in the first trimester can make administering cART to pregnant women challenging.[41–43] Specific counseling should be provided to women about nausea and vomiting because missing doses or suboptimal absorption can lead to subtherapeutic levels and can lead to drug resistance.

Initial Evaluation

Initial evaluation of a pregnant woman with HIV should include thorough review of past medical history, HIV-related illnesses, and previous ARV treatment regimens if the patient was diagnosed prior to pregnancy as well as plasma HIV RNA levels, CD4 T-lymphocyte (CD4) cell counts, and review of prior laboratory results. In those with newly diagnosed HIV infection during pregnancy, determination of risk factors for HIV infection should be performed as well as partner history and partner notification with the assistance of available social workers, HIV counselors, or local public health departments. In addition, any problems with adherence or tolerance should be carefully considered. HIV genotyping/drug-resistance studies should be performed before initiating or changing cART regimens in pregnancy if a patient's viral load is above 500 to 1000 copies/mL. If HIV is initially diagnosed in the late second or third trimester, cART should be started immediately without awaiting resistance test results, with subsequent modification of therapy if necessary once those results return. The authors strongly recommend consultation with an HIV expert when beginning such an empiric regimen, with the Perinatal HIV/AIDS Clinician Consultation Center an excellent, no-cost resource for consultation. Screening for hepatitis C and tuberculosis in addition to the standard hepatitis B, syphilis, and gonorrhea/chlamydia screens should be performed as well as assessment of the need for prophylaxis against opportunistic infections.[40] As addressed previously, serologic screening for CMV and toxoplasmosis and symptomatic screening for vaginal infections are recommended. HSV seroscreening may also be considered in at-risk individuals. Finally, at the initial visit, vaccinations should also be addressed and administered per ACOG recommendations.[44,45]

cART in Pregnancy

The perinatal guidelines developed by the Department of Health and Human Services Office of AIDS Research Advisory Council have recently been revised and updated in

March 2014.[40] Pregnant women with HIV should be offered a cART regimen consisting of at least 3 drugs, with the selection of drugs dependent on whether the woman is treatment naïve, has demonstrated resistance to certain drugs, or has other toxicity considerations. In addition, drug selection should include a nucleoside reverse transcriptase inhibitor (NRTI) that crosses the placenta well to achieve pre-exposure prophylaxis for the fetus/infant. Current cART regimens outside of pregnancy are recommended to include 2 NRTIs/nucleotide reverse transcriptase inhibitors (NtRTIs) plus a third agent from either the PI, non-NRTI (NNRTI), or integrase inhibitor drug classes. Although zidovudine no longer is first-line therapy for nonpregnant patients, it remains a preferred agent for use in pregnancy given its tested ability to cross the placenta and prevent perinatal HIV transmission.[46]

The evidence reviewed in the perinatal guidelines suggests that the pharmacokinetics of NRTIs/NtRTIs/NNRTIs are not affected greatly by the physiologic changes of pregnancy. The pharmacokinetics of PIs, however, seem more vulnerable to the effects of pregnancy, especially in the third trimester, and may require checking plasma levels with level-indicated or empiric dose adjustments.[40]

Teratogenicity is always a concern for medication administration during pregnancy. All pregnant women who receive ARVs during pregnancy should be reported to the Antiretroviral Pregnancy Registry. Efavirenz merits special consideration, however, because it has been associated with an increased risk of neural tube defects in some studies but not others.[36,47,48] These studies are hampered by low numbers and recall bias; thus, further study is warranted. Prospective studies do not demonstrate an increased signal for anomalies. The current guidelines recommend women receiving efavirenz should be practicing good contraception to avoid pregnancy, and this drug should be avoided in the first 8 weeks of pregnancy.[49,50]

Studies suggest that early, sustained suppression of HIV viral load is associated with decreased risk of perinatal transmission. Long-term risks posed to the fetus by first-trimester ARV exposure, however, are not fully known. In addition, first-trimester nausea and vomiting may make medication compliance difficult. Providers should take these factors as well as patient HIV disease status into consideration. In some women, delaying initiation of therapy until after 12 weeks may be reasonable. After 12 weeks' gestation, cART therapy should be started as soon as possible regardless of viral load to decrease the risk of perinatal transmission.[40]

Discontinuation or changing ARV regimens that are effectively suppressing viral load is not recommended. Specifically, efavirenz does not need to be discontinued because most pregnancies are not confirmed until after the neural tube is closed at 5 to 6 weeks' gestation. Additionally, a recent publication found that interruption of ARV during pregnancy[51] was associated with an increased risk for perinatal transmission[51] and loss of virologic control, which may consequently increase risks for perinatal transmission.[49] Hyperemesis gravidarum and nausea and vomiting of pregnancy should be aggressively managed so that missed doses or nonabsorbed doses of ART do not promote viral resistance. If ART medications need to be stopped, then expert consultation is recommended, particularly when NNRTIs are used, given their prolonged half-life compared with other ART classes.[40,52]

Although there seems to be an increased risk for adverse pregnancy outcomes in women with untreated HIV, there has been conflicting evidence as to whether cART increases the risk for preterm birth (PTB). There may be a small increased risk for PTB in particular using PI-based cART; however, when a recent study controlled for multiple factors, such as HIV disease stage, types of ART, and medical and obstetric complications, PI-based cART was not more associated with spontaneous PTB than non-PI–based cART.[53] Injection drug use and more advanced disease in a recent meta-analysis remain risk factors with increased rates of PTB.[54] The potential small increased risk for PTB is outweighed by the benefits of cART and PI-based therapy to prevent perinatal transmission.[40]

Treatment regimens should be prescribed in a manner to ensure maximal adherence and future treatment options. This means considering factors, such as patient convenience and limiting the pill burden, with combined dosage, patient comorbidities, potential side effects that may be worsened in pregnancy, and potential interactions with other medications. The importance of strict adherence to the prescribed regimen should be stressed to patients to prevent the development of drug resistance (**Table 1**).[8,40]

Table 1, adapted from the perinatal guidelines, suggests which drug combinations to start in drug-naïve women. These usually include a 2-drug NRTI backbone plus either a ritonavir-boosted PI or non-nucleoside analog (NNRTI). For reasons discussed previously, efavirenz should not be started in the first trimester before 8 weeks' gestation. For further details on management of HIV and antiretroviral therapy in pregnancy, please see the **Box 1**. For ARV experienced women, consultation with a HIV specialist is recommended if the patient is not already on a successful ARV regimen.

MODE OF DELIVERY

Prior to the era when cART was universally recommended in pregnancy, a multicenter randomized clinical trial established that the perinatal HIV transmission rate was 1.8% in infants born by scheduled cesarean section versus 10.5% born vaginally,[60] and a subsequent meta-analysis of 15 prospective cohort studies demonstrated a 50% reduction in perinatal transmission with scheduled cesarean delivery compared with vaginal delivery.[61] These studies were performed, however, before women routinely received cART during pregnancy and had no viral load information to guide delivery planning. Therefore, data from these studies and another study documenting no cases of perinatal transmission in 57 women with viral load less than or equal to 1000 copies/mL[62] were used as indirect evidence to guide ACOG to recommend the use of the level of 1000 copies/mL as that at which patients should be counseled on the potential benefits of scheduled cesarean to lower risk of perinatal transmission during delivery.[63] Subsequent studies done in the era of cART have shown perinatal transmission can occur at viral loads less than 1000 copies/mL. These rates, however,

Table 1 Recommendations for ARV use during pregnancy in the treatment-naïve patient	
Preferred Two-NRTI Backbone	Abacavir[a] + Lamivudine Tenofovir[b] + Emtricitabine or Tenofovir + Lamivudine Zidovudine + Lamivudine[c]
Protease Inhibitor Regimen	Atazanavir/Ritonavir + a preferred two-NRTI backbone Lopinavir/Ritonavir + a preferred two-NRTI backbone
NNRTI Regimen	Efavirenz[d] + a preferred two-NRTI backbone

For ARV-naive women, a cART regimen including two NRTIs and either a PI with low-dose ritonavir or an NNRTI is preferable.
[a] Risk of hypersensitivity reaction, should only be given if patient tests negative for HLA-B5701.
[b] Tenofovir can be renal toxic, use with caution with patients with renal insufficiency.
[c] Most experience for use during pregnancy, can have hematologic toxicity.
[d] Initiate after 8 week of gestation due to concerns for teratogenicity.
Adapted from Panel on Treatment of HIV-Infected Pregnant Women and Prevention of Perinatal Transmission. Recommendations for use of antiretroviral drugs in pregnant HIV-1- infected women for maternal health and interventions to reduce perinatal HIV transmission in the United States. Available at: http://aidsinfo.nih.gov/guidelines/html/3/perinatal-guidelines/0/.

Box 1
Monitoring during pregnancy

- Viral load: initial visit, 2–4 weeks after starting or changing ARV drugs and then monthly until undetectable, then q 3 months until delivery. Should also be checked at 34–36 weeks for delivery planning and for planning neonatal drug therapy.

- CD4 count: initial visit, then q 3 months (q 6 months if undetectable viral load and low risk for opportunistic infections).

- Genotypic ARV drug-resistance testing: perform prior to starting drug therapy (so simultaneously if second/third trimester) if viral load greater than 500–1000 copies/mL or if cART is started and viral load is not suppressed.

- Monitoring for ARV drug complications dependent on maternal drug regimen (ie, liver function tests if on PI, renal function if on tenofovir, complete blood cell count if on nucleoside analog [see http://aidsinfo.nih.gov/contentfiles/lvguidelines/PerinatalGL.pdf for further details on specific agents]).

- Standard gestational diabetes screening at 24–28 weeks or earlier if they have additional risk factors for gestational DM. Some experts recommend early screening if on chronic PI therapy given association between PI therapy and hyperglycemia.[55]

- First-trimester ultrasound for accurate dating to guide delivery planning.

- Amniocentesis: reserve for obstetric indications. Before cART, invasive procedures, including chorionic villus sampling and amniocentesis, were associated with 2- to 4-fold increase in risk of perinatal HIV transmission.[56] In women with low viral loads on cART, however, invasive procedures do not seem to increase this risk although they cannot be ruled out entirely.[57] Therefore, the expert consensus is to obtain optimal viral suppression and if possible to avoid the placenta during the procedure and to consider use of cell-free fetal DNA testing to avoid amniocentesis when possible.[58]

- Antepartum fetal surveillance is not specifically recommended for pregnancies complicated by HIV infection. Comorbidities are often present and surveillance is recommended, however, based on the comorbidities as outlined by the National Institute of Child Health and Human Development and ACOG.[59] Patients with suspected or known primary HIV infection during pregnancy, late pregnancy initiation of ART, or use of newer agents for which there is little pregnancy experience represent clinical scenarios where providers might recommend antenatal surveillance.

Adapted from Panel on Treatment of HIV-Infected Pregnant Women and Prevention of Perinatal Transmission. Recommendations for use of antiretroviral drugs in pregnant HIV-1-infected women for maternal health and interventions to reduce perinatal HIV transmission in the United States. Available at: http://aidsinfo.nih.gov/guidelines/html/3/perinatal-guidelines/0/.

---

are low—1.2% overall, regardless of mode of delivery in the European Collaborative Study,[34] and there have been no data to show that scheduled cesarean decreases the perinatal transmission rate in women treated with cART throughout pregnancy with consistent viral loads less than or equal to 1000 copies/mL.[40]

It is recommended that women with viral loads greater than or equal to 1000 copies/mL or with unknown viral loads be offered scheduled cesarean section delivery at 38 weeks' gestation to maximally decrease the risk of perinatal transmission.[40] Guidelines for elective delivery given to the uncomplicated obstetric population to prevent complications of iatrogenic prematurity suggest waiting until 39 weeks.[64] The benefit in preventing perinatal HIV transmission associated with labor/rupture of membranes by performing planned cesarean sections at 38 weeks is generally accepted to outweigh the risk of iatrogenic prematurity incurred by delivery a week earlier. If a cesarean section is planned for an obstetric indication (ie, elective repeat cesarean or malpresentation), however, and not to decrease perinatal HIV transmission, it should be scheduled for 39 weeks.[63]

It is unclear if performing cesarean section in women with viral loads greater than or equal to 1000 copies/mL after labor onset or rupture of membranes decreases perinatal HIV transmission. One meta-analysis of women with HIV on zidovudine or no ARV medication showed a 2% increased risk of perinatal transmission associated with each additional hour that membranes were ruptured prior to delivery.[65] Other studies comparing HIV-infected women who have rupture of membranes or labor and then undergo cesarean section for obstetric indications, however, versus women who deliver vaginally showed no difference in perinatal transmission rates.[66] Therefore, mode of delivery decisions to prevent HIV transmission in these cases should be individualized and take into account factors, such as viral load, duration of membrane rupture, amount of time expected until vaginal delivery, and current ARV therapy. Regardless of the delivery route chosen, a patient's current ARV therapy should be continued and IV zidovudine administered if viral load is unknown or greater than or equal to 1000 copies/mL (discussed later).[40]

INTRAPARTUM CARE

Intrapartum ARV therapy is dictated by the ARV regimen a pregnant woman has received during pregnancy and the degree of viral suppression that has been achieved. According to the perinatal guidelines, women on cART antepartum should continue their established drug regimen as much as possible during labor or prior to having a scheduled cesarean section.[40]

Based on evidence from several large cohort studies, if an HIV-infected woman has been receiving and adherent to cART in late pregnancy and has consistently had an HIV viral load less than or equal to 1000 copies/mL, then it is not necessary to administer IV zidovudine during labor/prior to cesarean to prevent perinatal transmission. Previously, it had been recommended to do so if the maternal viral load was not less than or equal to 400 copies/mL; however, more recent evidence has shown that this limit can be safely liberalized to 1000 copies/mL.[67] Zidovudine administration intrapartum for women with viral loads greater than or equal to 1000 copies/mL is still recommended even if previous zidovudine resistance has been identified, because it is still thought to be of benefit to prevent perinatal transmission.[40] If viral load has not consistently been below 1000 copies/mL in late pregnancy or if there is concern about medication adherence, it is left to a clinician's judgment to use zidovudine intrapartum to prevent perinatal transmission.[40]

Women who present in labor and have no documented HIV test result in pregnancy should be screened with rapid HIV testing. If these results are positive, they should be assumed to be HIV infected and treatment initiated without delay for confirmatory testing with immediate initiation of IV zidovudine therapy. Consultation with an HIV specialist is recommended in this circumstance for additional recommendations for treatment of mother and infant.

Intrapartum management should avoid anything that may increase potential perinatal transmission. These include labor interventions, such as artificial rupture of membranes, use of intrauterine pressure catheters or fetal scalp electrodes, or operative vaginal delivery via vacuum or forceps.[8]

For postpartum hemorrhage, use of methylergonovine is discouraged in women on ART. Agents known to inhibit cytochrome P450 3A4 (CYP3A4) enzyme inhibitors, such as PIs, have been linked with dangerous hypertension. Other ART agents, however, are CYP3A4 inducers, such as the NNRTI (eg, nevirapine and efavirenz), and have the potential for decreasing methylergonovine levels resulting in lower efficacy.

In this setting, oxytocin, misoprostol, and prostaglandin F2α are better choices for pharmacologic management of postpartum hemorrhage.[40]

POSTPARTUM ISSUES

If ARV therapy is newly initiated during pregnancy, then continuation versus discontinuation of ART postpartum ideally should be discussed during pregnancy. Evidence for continuation of ART for maternal health exists for those with CD4 count less than 350 cells/mm^3, those with CD4 counts 350 to 550 cells/mm^3, and those with CD4 greater than 550 cells/mm^3, although the strength of evidence to continue is better at lower CD4 count categories. The decision is complex because the postpartum period presents additional challenges for medication adherence. Linkage to HIV care if HIV is newly diagnosed in pregnancy or a patient was not previously linked to HIV care and other support services also ideally should be established during pregnancy and certainly by hospital discharge.

When ARV medications are discontinued, special attention should be paid if a patient is receiving a NNRTI, such as nevirapine or efavirenz. These medications have a long half-life and can be detected up to 21 days or even longer after discontinuation, predisposing to subtherapeutic drug levels and NNRTI-resistant mutations. Although the optimal duration of other ART continuation has not been clearly defined, 7 to 30 days of continuation or substituting a PI plus 2 other agents has been suggested.[40]

Breastfeeding

Because of the continued risk for transmission of HIV to neonates/infants through breast milk, breastfeeding in resource-rich nations is strongly discouraged. In low-resource nations, breastfeeding is recommended due to the lack of clean water for formula and increased risk of mortality from other infections. In the recent Breastfeeding, Antiretrovirals and Nutrition trial, maternal and infant ARV decrease the risk of breastfeeding-associated transmission to 1.7% from 5.7%.[68] Mixed breastfeeding and bottle-feeding is also associated with increased risks of HIV transmission compared with exclusive breastfeeding. Because of stigma associated with HIV, many HIV-infected women have not disclosed their infection to family and friends. In many societies where HIV is endemic, lack of breastfeeding is assumed to mean the mother is HIV infected. Thus, to appease friends and family members' suspicion, breastfeeding may be contemplated. Additionally, HIV-infected women in resource-rich nations, such as the United States, are conflicted by public health and other campaigns promoting "breast is best." For at least these reasons, investigating the personal beliefs and familial and cultural traditions surrounding breastfeeding for all HIV-infected gravidas is paramount to understanding the emotional conflict about this issue and allowing care providers to minimize the risk of perinatal transmission of HIV from undisclosed exclusive or intermittent breastfeeding. With cART and undetectable serum viral load, the risk for breastfeeding transmission of HIV is very low but not zero and is still not recommended. A recently published thoughtful review offers a script for HIV-infected gravidas to address and validate their desires and motivations, discuss alternatives to breastfeeding, and develops a harm reduction approach and evidence-based protocol for women who still prefer to breastfeed.[69]

Other Infant Feeding Practices

Premastication (chewing of food before giving it to an infant/toddler) is also discouraged because this has been identified as a factor for transmission of HIV and needs to be specifically discussed.[70]

CARE OF HUMAN IMMUNODEFICIENCY VIRUS-EXPOSED NEONATE

Chemoprophylaxis with 4 to 6 weeks of zidovudine is generally recommended for HIV-exposed neonates. Additional medications may be recommended for prophylaxis in high-risk neonates, for instance those with with suboptimally controlled disease antepartum who did not receive optimal intrapartum dosing.[40] Additional material about infant ARV prophylaxis is available in the perinatal guidelines and from Perinatal HIV/AIDS Clinician Consultation Center.

Suggested infant HIV testing schedule and when testing is considered negative are also available in the perinatal guidelines. According to these guidelines, if there are 2 or more negative tests (nucleic acid testing, including DNA or RNA polymerase chain reaction), with one at age 14 days or older and a second at more than 1 month of age, HIV can be reasonably excluded. This expedited time frame of testing allows for reassurance to mothers and their families. Definitive exclusion of HIV infection in an infant depends on 2 negative virologic tests with one performed at greater than 1 month of age and the second at greater than 4 months of age. Many experts recommend an HIV antibody test at or after 12 to 18 months of age. Because maternal HIV antibodies cross the placenta and persist in the infant for many months, HIV antibody testing is not recommended before 12 months of age because positive tests may reflect persistent maternal antibodies rather than an infant's antibody response to infection.[40]

CONTRACEPTION

At the time of routine clinical care visits for nonpregnant women and gynecologic visits, reproductive desires should be addressed (Appendix B). For those not interested in pregnancy or those whose medical conditions should be optimized prior to conception, contraception should be discussed. Those living with HIV should have access to all methods of contraception.

Barrier contraception is advised for all acts of sexual intercourse for prevention of HIV to sexual partners. Hormonal methods of contraception, primarily oral contraceptive pills, are associated with the possibility for significant interactions with ARV therapy. The HIV perinatal guidelines extensively revised their summary of the literature on this subject and formed a consensus on which alterations to make in hormonal contraception with individualized ARV agents. A detailed chart of the expert panel's consensus is available at http://aidsinfo.nih.gov/guidelines/html/3/perinatal-guidelines/152/overview.

Alternative methods of contraception are recommended when efavirenz or nevirapine (NNRTIs) or boosted PIs as well as some unboosted PIs are used with either oral contraceptive pills (combined oral contraceptives or progestin-only pills) or hormonal implants are used. Other forms of contraception can be used provided no other contraindications exist. HIV is not a contraindication to intrauterine device (IUD) use.[71] Given potential for adherence issues, pill burden, and other social issues, long-acting contraceptive methods may be more successful. Emergency contraception should also be prescribed as appropriate for an ARV regimen. More information about emergency contraception and HIV is available in the *A Guide to the Clinical Care of Women with HIV/AIDS*.[8]

SUMMARY

New developments in pharmacologic management of HIV make it difficult for obstetricians to keep abreast with the recommended regimens. The field has progressed, however, such that perinatal transmission of the HIV virus is almost entirely preventable if the proper management strategies are used.

Three Web sites should be bookmarked on a computer to assist when HIV and pregnancy arises:

1. http://aidsinfo.nih.gov/contentfiles/lvguidelines/PerinatalGL.pdf for access to the Department of Health and Human Services Office of AIDS Research Advisory Council perinatal guidelines. Available free of charge online and updated frequently.
2. www.hab.hrsa.gov for access to *A Guide to the Clinical Care of Women with HIV/AIDS*. Available free of charge online and updated frequently.
3. The National Clinical Consultation Center Perinatal HIV/AIDS Consultation Service, National Clinical Consultation Center at University of California San Francisco is available through the University of California, San Francisco, is available at 1-888-448-8765 and at nccc.ucsf.edu to help when clinical scenarios arise in which specialized assistance/consultation is necessary either for diagnosis and treatment of HIV/AIDS in pregnancy, or for preconception or contraceptive management.

REFERENCES

1. Hare B. Clinical overview of HIV disease. Introduction and history. Available at: http://www.hivinsite.ucsf.edu. Accessed May 14, 2014.
2. Mofenson L. Protecting the next generation—eliminating perinatal HIV-1 infection. N Engl J Med 2010;362:2316–8.
3. Nesheim S, Taylor A, Lampe MA, et al. A framework for elimination of perinatal transmission of HIV in the United States. Pediatrics 2012;130(4):1–7.
4. Nesheim S, Harris LF, Lampe M. Elimination of perinatal HIV infection in the USA and other high income countries: achievements and challenges. Curr Opin HIV AIDS 2013;8(5):447–56.
5. Available at: http://www.medpagetoday.com/InfectiousDisease/PublicHealth/17594. Accessed May 14, 2014.
6. Hare B. Clinical overview of HIV disease, transmission and risk factors. Available at: http://www.hivinsite.ucsf.edu. Accessed May 14, 2014.
7. Centers for Disease Control and Prevention (CDC). Revised surveillance case definition for HIV infection—United States, 2014. MMWR Recomm Rep 2014; 63(RR-03):1–10.
8. US Dept of Health and Human Services, Health Resources and Services. A guide to the clinical care of women with HIV/AIDS—2013 edition. Rockville (MD): US Department of Health and Human Services; 2013. Available at: http://www.hab.hrsa.gov.
9. Available at: http://www.unaids.org/en/resrouces/campaigns/globalreport2013/factsheet. Accessed April 15, 2014.
10. Available at: http://www.cdc.gov/hiv/statistics/basics/ataglance.html. Accessed April 15, 2014.
11. Available at: http://www.cdc.gov/hiv/pdf/statistics_surveillance_Women.pdf. Accessed April 16, 2014.
12. HIV among pregnant women, infants, and children in the United States. Available at: http://www.cdc.gov/hiv/pdf/risk_WIC.pdf. Accessed May 14, 2014.
13. Kourtis AP, Bulterys M. Mother-to-child transmission of HIV: pathogenesis, mechanisms and pathways. Clin Perinatol 2010;37(4):721–37.
14. Panel on Antiretroviral Guidelines for Adults and Adolescents. Guidelines for the use of antiretroviral agents in HIV-1-infected adults and adolescents. Department of Health and Human Services. Acute and Recent (Early) HIV Infection, I1–5. Available at: http://aidsinfo.nih.gov/ContentFiles/AdultandAdolescentGL.pdf. Accessed June 1, 2014.

15. Singh S, Lampe MA, Surendera B, et al. HIV seroconversion during pregnancy and mother-to-child HIV transmission: data from the enhanced perinatal surveillance projects, United States, 2005–2010. Paper presented at: 20th Conference on Retroviruses and Opportunistic Infections (CROI 2013). Atlanta (GA), March 3-7, 2013.

16. Lampe MA, Smith DK, Anderson GJ, et al. Achieving safe conception in HIV-discordant couples: the potential role of oral preexposure prophylaxis (PrEP) in the United States. Am J Obstet Gynecol 2011;204(6):488.e1–8.

17. Koenig LJ, Espinoza L, Hodge K, et al. Young, seropositive, and pregnant: epidemiologic and psychosocial perspectives on pregnant adolescents with human immunodeficiency virus infection. Am J Obstet Gynecol 2007;197(3 Suppl):S123–31.

18. Floridia M, Tamburrini E, Ravizza M, et al. Antiretroviral therapy at conception in pregnant women with HIV in Italy: wide range of variability and frequent exposure to contraindicated drugs. Antivir Ther 2006;11(7):941–6.

19. Savasi V, Mandia L, Laoreti A, et al. Reproductive assistance in HIV serodiscordant couples. Hum Reprod Update 2013;19(2):136–50.

20. Lambert JS, Watts DH, Mofenson L, et al. Risk factors for preterm birth, low birth weight, and intrauterine growth retardation in infants born to HIV-infected pregnant women receiving zidovudine. Pediatric AIDS Clinical Trials Group 185 Team. AIDS 2000;14(10):1389–99.

21. Mugo NR, Heffron R, Donnell D, et al. Increased risk of HIV-1 transmission in pregnancy: a prospective study among African HIV-1-serodiscordant couples. AIDS 2011;25(15):1887–95.

22. Xu F, Sternberg MR, Kottiri BJ, et al. Trends in herpes simplex virus type 1 and type 2 seroprevalence in the United States. JAMA 2006;296(8):964–73.

23. Chen KT, Segu M, Lumey LH, et al. Genital herpes simplex virus infection and perinatal transmission of human immunodeficiency virus. Obstet Gynecol 2005;106(6):1341–8.

24. ACOG Committee on Practice Bulletins. ACOG Practice Bulletin. Clinical management guidelines for obstetrician-gynecologists. No. 82 June 2007. Management of herpes in pregnancy. Obstet Gynecol 2007;109(6):1489–98.

25. Thomas SL, Newell ML, Peckham CS, et al. A review of hepatitis C virus (HCV) vertical transmission: risks of transmission to infants born to mothers with and without HCV viraemia or human immunodeficiency virus infection. Int J Epidemiol 1998;27(1):108–17.

26. Mast EE, Hwang LY, Seto DS, et al. Risk factors for perinatal transmission of hepatitis C virus (HCV) and the natural history of HCV infection acquired in infancy. J Infect Dis 2005;192(11):1880–9.

27. Alter MJ. Epidemiology of viral hepatitis and HIV co-infection. J Hepatol 2006; 44(1 Suppl):S6–9.

28. Mavenyengwa RT, Moyo SR, Nordbo SA. Streptococcus agalactiae colonization and correlation with HIV-1 and HBV seroprevalence in pregnant women from Zimbabwe. Eur J Obstet Gynecol Reprod Biol 2010;150(1):34–8.

29. Breese P, Burman W, Shlay J, et al. The effectiveness of a verbal opt-out system for human immunodeficiency virus screening during pregnancy. Obstet Gynecol 2004;104(1):134–7.

30. One Test Two Lives Fact Sheet. Reducing HIV transmission from mother-to-child: an opt-out approach to HIV screening. Atlanta (GA): Centers for Disease Control and Prevention (CDC); 2008.

31. Office of the Inspector General. Reducing obstetrician barriers to offering HIV testing. Washington, DC: Department of Health and Human Services; 2002.

32. Royce RA, Walter EB, Fernandez MI, et al. Barriers to universal prenatal HIV testing in 4 US locations in 1997. Am J Public Health 2001;91(5):727–33.
33. DRAFT Recommendations: diagnostic laboratory testing for HIV infection in the United States. In CDC 2012 HIV Diagnostics Conference Feedback Session. December 14, 2012.
34. European Collaborative Study. Mother-to-child transmission of HIV infection in the era of highly active antiretroviral therapy. Clin Infect Dis 2005;40(3):458–65.
35. Tubiana R, Le Chenadec J, Rouzioux C, et al. Factors associated with mother-to-child transmission of HIV-1 despite a maternal viral load <500 copies/ml at delivery: a case-control study nested in the French perinatal cohort (EPF-ANRS CO1). Clin Infect Dis 2010;50(4):585–96.
36. Warszawski J, Tubiana R, Le Chenadec J, et al. Mother-to-child HIV transmission despite antiretroviral therapy in the ANRS French Perinatal Cohort. AIDS 2008;22(2):289–99.
37. Cu-Uvin S, Caliendo AM. Genital tract HIV-1 RNA shedding among women with below detectable plasma viral load. AIDS 2011;25(6):880–1.
38. Cu-Uvin S, DeLong AK, Venkatesh KK, et al. Genital tract HIV-1 RNA shedding among women with below detectable plasma viral load. AIDS 2010;24(16): 2489–97.
39. Antiretroviral Pregnancy Registry Steering Committee. Antiretroviral pregnancy registry International Interim report for 1 January 1989 through 31 July 2013. Wilmington (NC): Registry Coordinating Center; 2013. Available at: http://www. APRegistry.com.
40. Panel on Treatment of HIV-Infected Pregnant Women and Prevention of Perinatal Transmission. Recommendations for use of antiretroviral drugs in pregnant HIV-1-infected women for maternal health and interventions to reduce perinatal HIV transmission in the United States. Available at: http://aidsinfo.nih.gov/contentfiles/lvguidelines/PerinatalGL.pdf. Accessed April 1, 2014.
41. Minkoff H, Augenbraun M. Antiretroviral therapy for pregnant women. Am J Obstet Gynecol 1997;176(2):478–89.
42. Mirochnick M, Capparelli E. Pharmacokinetics of antiretrovirals in pregnant women. Clin Pharmacokinet 2004;43(15):1071–87.
43. Roustit M, Jlaiel M, Leclercq P, et al. Pharmacokinetics and therapeutic drug monitoring of antiretrovirals in pregnant women. Br J Clin Pharmacol 2008; 66(2):179–95.
44. ACOG Committee Opinion No. 566: update on immunization and pregnancy: tetanus, diphtheria, and pertussis vaccination. Obstet Gynecol 2013;121:1411–4.
45. American College of Obstetricians and Gynecologists Committee on Obstetric Practice. ACOG Committee Opinion No. 468: influenza vaccination during pregnancy. Obstet Gynecol 2010;116:1006–7.
46. Connor EM, Sperling RS, Gelber R, et al. Reduction of maternal-infant transmission of human immunodeficiency virus type 1 with zidovudine treatment. Pediatric AIDS Clinical Trials Group Protocol 076 Study Group. N Engl J Med 1994; 331(18):1173–80.
47. Ford N, Calmy A, Mofenson L. Safety of efavirenz in the first trimester of pregnancy: an updated systematic review and meta-analysis. AIDS 2011;25(18):2301–4.
48. Watts DH. Teratogenicity risk of antiretroviral therapy in pregnancy. Curr HIV/AIDS Rep 2007;4(3):135–40.
49. Floridia M, Ravizza M, Pinnetti C, et al. Treatment change in pregnancy is a significant risk factor for detectable HIV-1 RNA in plasma at end of pregnancy. HIV Clin Trials 2010;11(6):303–11.

50. Venkatesh KK, DeLong AK, Kantor R, et al. Persistent genital tract HIV-1 RNA shedding after change in treatment regimens in antiretroviral-experienced women with detectable plasma viral load. J Womens Health (Larchmt) 2013; 22(4):330–8.
51. Galli L, Puliti D, Chiappini E, et al. Is the interruption of antiretroviral treatment during pregnancy an additional major risk factor for mother-to-child transmission of HIV type 1? Clin Infect Dis 2009;48(9):1310–7.
52. Committee on Practice Bulletins—Obstetrics, The American College of Obstetricians and Gynecologists. Practice bulletin no. 130: prediction and prevention of preterm birth. Obstet Gynecol 2012;120(4):964–73.
53. Patel K, Shapiro DE, Brogly SB, et al. Prenatal protease inhibitor use and risk of preterm birth among HIV-infected women initiating antiretroviral drugs during pregnancy. J Infect Dis 2010;201(7):1035–44.
54. Townsend C, Schulte J, Thorne C, et al. Antiretroviral therapy and preterm delivery-a pooled analysis of data from the United States and Europe. BJOG 2010;117(11):1399–410.
55. Food and Drug Administration. FDA Public Health Advisory: reports of diabetes and hyperglycemia in patients receiving protease inhibitors for treatment of human immunodeficiency virus (HIV). Rockville (MD): Food and Drug Administration; Public Health Service; Department of Health and Human Services; 1997. Available at: http://www.fda.gov/cder/news/proteaseletter.htm.
56. Shapiro DE, Sperling RS, Mandelbrot L, et al. Risk factors for perinatal human immunodeficiency virus transmission in patients receiving zidovudine prophylaxis. Pediatric AIDS Clinical Trials Group protocol 076 Study Group. Obstet Gynecol 1999;94(6):897–908.
57. Mandelbrot L, Jasseron C, Ekoukou D, et al. Amniocentesis and mother-to-child human immunodeficiency virus transmission in the Agence Nationale de Recherches sur le SIDA et les Hepatites Virales French Perinatal Cohort. Am J Obstet Gynecol 2009;200(2):160.e1–9.
58. American College of Obstetricians and Gynecologists Committee on Genetics. Committee Opinion No. 545: Non-invasive prenatal testing for fetal aneuploidy. Obstet Gynecol 2012;545:1–3.
59. Signore C, Freeman RK, Spong CY. Antenatal testing-a reevaluation: executive summary of a Eunice Kennedy Shriver National Institute of Child Health and Human Development workshop. Obstet Gynecol 2009;113(3): 687–701.
60. European Mode of Delivery Collaboration. Elective caesarean-section versus vaginal delivery in prevention of vertical HIV-1 transmission: a randomised clinical trial. Lancet 1999;353(9158):1035–9.
61. The mode of delivery and the risk of vertical transmission of human immunodeficiency virus type 1-a meta-analysis of 15 prospective cohort studies. The International Perinatal HIV Group. N Engl J Med 1999;340(13):977–87.
62. Garcia PM, Kalish LA, Pitt J, et al. Maternal levels of plasma human immunodeficiency virus type 1 RNA and the risk of perinatal transmission. Women and Infants Transmission Study Group. N Engl J Med 1999;341(6):394–402.
63. Committee on Obstetric Practice. ACOG committee opinion scheduled Cesarean delivery and the prevention of vertical transmission of HIV infection. Number 234, May 2000 (replaces number 219, August 1999). Int J Gynaecol Obstet 2001;73(3):279–81.
64. Tita AT, Landon MB, Spong CY, et al. Timing of elective repeat cesarean delivery at term and neonatal outcomes. N Engl J Med 2009;360(2):111–20.

65. International Perinatal HIV Group. Duration of ruptured membranes and vertical transmission of HIV-1: a meta-analysis from 15 prospective cohort studies. AIDS 2001;15(3):357–68.
66. Townsend CL, Cortina-Borja M, Peckham CS, et al. Low rates of mother-to-child transmission of HIV following effective pregnancy interventions in the United Kingdom and Ireland, 2000-2006. AIDS 2008;22(8):973–81.
67. Briand N, Warszawski J, Mandelbrot L, et al. Is intrapartum intravenous zidovudine for prevention of mother-to-child HIV-1 transmission still useful in the combination antiretroviral therapy era? Clin Infect Dis 2013;57(6):903–14.
68. Chasela CS, Hudgens MG, Jamieson DJ, et al. Maternal or infant antiretroviral drugs to reduce HIV-1 transmission. N Engl J Med 2010;362(24):2271–81.
69. Levison J, Weber S, Cohan D. Breastfeeding and human immunodeficiency virus-positive women in the United States: harm reduction counseling strategies. Clin Infect Dis 2014;59:304–9.
70. Ivy W 3rd, Dominguez KL, Rakhmanina NY, et al. Premastication as a route of pediatric HIV transmission: case-control and cross-sectional investigations. J Acquir Immune Defic Syndr 2012;59(2):207–12.
71. Browne H, Manipalviratn S, Armstrong A. Using an intrauterine device in immunocompromised women. Obstet Gynecol 2008;112(3):667–9.

APPENDIX A

HIV and Pregnancy: Decision Aids for the Patient and Provider

1. Patient Decision Aid

With effective HIV treatment, women and men with HIV infection can now enjoy a long and healthy life and can look forward to a future that may include planning a family. When taken during pregnancy, HIV medications can decrease the risk of transmitting HIV to the baby to 1%–2% or less. It is also important to prevent pregnancy when you are not yet ready to become a mother. As a woman with HIV, it is important to plan carefully so that you can get the treatment you need to have a safer pregnancy, prevent transmission of HIV to your baby, and prevent pregnancy until you are ready. This survey is designed to help you and your healthcare provider take the first steps in that planning.

Name: ——————————————— Date: —————

1. Your current age is —————

2. Have you ever been pregnant? ☐ **YES** ☐ **NO**

3. If **YES,** how many times? ————— How many children do you
   have? —————

4. Are you interested in getting pregnant? ☐ **YES** ☐ **NO**

5. If **YES,** when do you wish to conceive?
   ☐ Trying to conceive now ☐ 6 months – 1 year from now
   ☐ 1 – 2 years from now ☐ More than 2 years from now

6. Have you had sex with a man in the last 6 months? ☐ **YES** ☐ **NO**

7. Are you currently using condoms? ☐ **YES** ☐ **NO**

8. Are you currently using birth control other than condoms?

   A. What type?
      ☐ None ☐ Birth control pill ☐ IUD ☐ Injection (Depo-Provera)
      ☐ Patch/vaginal ring ☐ Implant under the skin (Implanon)
      ☐ Sterilization (tubes tied) ☐ Unsure
      ☐ Other: ————————————————

   B. Are you trying to get pregnant? ☐ **YES** ☐ **NO**

9. Would you or your partner like to talk to someone about planning a safer pregnancy that may reduce the risk of HIV transmission to your baby? ☐ **YES** ☐ **NO**

HIV and Pregnancy: Decision Aids for the Patient and Provider

2. Provider Decision Aid

This tool is designed to help you, the health care provider, better address fertility issues (desire to conceive and desire to prevent pregnancy) with your patients.

1. Patient is postmenopausal or post-hysterectomy.
   - A. Yes – End of tool
   - B. No – Go to question 2

2. Does patient wish to have more children?
   - A. Yes – Go to question 3
   - B. No – Go to question 5

3. Does patient wish to conceive within the next year?
   - A. Yes – Go to question 4
   - B. No – Go to question 5

4. Patient would like to conceive within the next year.
   - A. Review medication list with patient for drugs that are contraindicated in women trying to conceive (eg, efavirenz, statins, ribavarin, tetracycline/ doxycycline). Other drugs should be used unless no alternate agents are available that are both effective and safer in women who are trying to conceive.

   AND
   - B. Offer and encourage referral for preconception counseling and evaluation.

5. Patient wishes to prevent pregnancy.
   - A. Patient has completed childbearing: refer to a gynecologist to discuss long-term or permanent options for contraception.

   OR
   - B. Patient wants more children but not within the next year: review nonpermanent options for contraception and strongly recommend referral for preconception counseling.

Key Considerations:

1. Patient has a problem with irregular menses or amenorrhea: if yes, perform a pregnancy test and refer for a gynecologic evaluation.
2. Menopause: can be difficult to diagnose
   - If the woman is >50 y with no vaginal bleeding for >1 y, she is postmenopausal.
   - If uncertain, refer for a gynecologic evaluation.
3. Formal preconception counseling and evaluation are strongly recommended if the patient
   - A. Is in a serodiscordant relationship
   - B. Has significant medical comorbidities
   - C. Has problems with substance abuse
   - D. Is taking a medication that is contraindicated in women trying to conceive
   - E. Reports a desire to conceive and a history of infertility or difficulty getting pregnant

APPENDIX B

Evaluation

Outlines the comprehensive preconception evaluation designed to identify factors that may affect a woman's ability to get pregnant or may increase the risk of adverse pregnancy outcomes for the mother or her fetus.

Comprehensive Preconception Evaluation	
History	**Comments**
HIV	• Date of diagnosis • History of OIs or other HIV-related illnesses • ART history, including use in prior pregnancies and/or reasons for change(s) in ART regimen (eg, adverse effects, resistance, tolerability) • Adherence history and challenges • Results of resistance tests • Nadir and current CD4$^+$ cell count • Current HIV VL
Pregnancy	• Number of previous pregnancies and their outcomes (eg, miscarriages, abortions, ectopic pregnancy, preterm births) • Number of living children and ages • Number of HIV-infected children • Pregnancy complications (eg, preterm laboratory, preeclampsia, birth defects) • Modes of delivery
Gynecologic	• Prior and current contraception use • Satisfaction with current contraception method and/or adverse effects • Current condom use and consistency of use (100% vs <100%) • Prior STIs or genital tract infections • Past difficulties in conceiving • Abnormal Pap smears and treatment • Other gynecologic problems and treatment (eg, fibroids, endometriosis)
General medical and surgical	• Other medical conditions (eg, DM, HTN, renal or cardiac disease, depression or other psychiatric illness) • All prior surgery • Blood type and history of transfusions • Allergies
Immunizations	• HBV, HAV, influenza, pneumococcus, HPV, tetanus
Medications	• All prescribed medications • All OTC medications • All complementary medications
Nutrition	• History of anemia or nutritional deficiencies • Special diet (eg, vegetarian, vegan, gluten-free) • Use of nutritional supplements and vitamins
Social history	• Relationship status • Use of illicit drugs, tobacco, alcohol • Employment status • Social support and disclosure to partner and others • Economic support • History and nature of domestic violence (ie, physical, sexual, psychological)

(continued on next page)

Table
(continued)

Comprehensive Preconception Evaluation	
History	**Comments**
Family history of heritable diseases	• Birth defects • Chromosomal abnormalities • Muscular dystrophy • Sickle cell disease • Mental retardation • Others

Male partner	• HIV status and knowledge of partner's status
	• If HIV-infected:
	  ○ Disclosure status
	  ○ History of OIs and other HIV-related conditions
	  ○ ART history and history of adverse effects, resistance, adherence problems
	  ○ Nadir and current CD4$^+$ cell count
	  ○ Current HIV VL
	• Medical and reproductive history
	• Medications
	• Use of illicit drugs, tobacco, alcohol
	• Employment status

Physical examination	• Comprehensive, with focus on genital tract
Laboratory (Emphasis is on lab tests that affect counseling and/or result in changes in care prior to pregnancy)	• Tests • STI screening: GC/chlamydia; syphilis; HSV culture or HSV-2 antibody, if indicated • CBC • Current CD4$^+$ cell count • HIV RNA • Resistance testing, if indicated • Rubella • HBV: HBsAb, HBsAg • HCV antibody and HCV RNA, if indicated • Pap smear • Other, as indicated by medical history and medications

Abbreviations: DM, Diabetes Mellitus; GC, Gonorrhea; HAV, Hepatitis A virus; HBsAb, Hepatitis B surface antibody; HBsAg, Hepatitis B surface antigen; HBV, Hepatitis B virus; HCV, Hepatitis C virus; HPV, Human papillomavirus; HTN, Hypertension; OI, Opportunistic infection; OTC, Over the counter; STI, Sexually transmitted infections; VL, Viral load.

Prevention and Management of Viral Hepatitis in Pregnancy

Martha W.F. Rac, MD*, Jeanne S. Sheffield, MD

KEYWORDS

- Hepatitis A • Hepatitis B • Hepatitis C • Hepatitis D • Hepatitis E • Viral hepatitis
- Pregnancy

KEY POINTS

- Hepatitis A virus infection is an acute self-limiting infection with a benign course during pregnancy.
- Hepatitis B virus (HBV) infection can cause both acute and chronic hepatitis. Although HBV does not seem to adversely affect pregnancy outcomes, vertical transmission is a risk that is significantly reduced by immunoprophylaxis of the newborn.
- Hepatitis C virus (HCV) infection is the most common blood-borne infection in the United States. Vertical transmission seems to be related to degree of maternal viremia, and efforts for vaccine development are promising.
- Hepatitis D virus (HDV) requires coinfection with HBV for propagation, and tends to have a more rapid progression to cirrhosis despite suppressing HBV viremia. Prevention of HBV is the mainstay of the prevention of HDV.
- Hepatitis E virus is the most common cause of acute hepatitis worldwide, and portends a 20% risk of maternal mortality during pregnancy. Two vaccines are available for at-risk populations in China, but studies are needed in pregnant populations before widespread use becomes viable.

HEPATITIS A
Introduction

Disease description

Hepatitis A virus (HAV) is a single-stranded 27-nm RNA picornavirus. HAV infection is usually a self-limiting illness that does not lead to chronic infection, and HAV immunoglobulin G (IgG) provides lifelong immunity. The average incubation period is 4 weeks. The virus can be detected in blood and feces 10 to 12 days after initial infection. A person is most contagious 14 to 21 days before the onset of symptoms and

The authors report no conflicts of interest.
Department of Obstetrics and Gynecology, University of Texas Southwestern Medical Center, 5323 Harry Hines Boulevard, Dallas, TX 75390-9032, USA
* Corresponding author.
E-mail address: Martha.Rac@utsouthwestern.edu

Obstet Gynecol Clin N Am 41 (2014) 573–592
http://dx.doi.org/10.1016/j.ogc.2014.08.004
0889-8545/14/$ – see front matter © 2014 Elsevier Inc. All rights reserved.

continues to be so 1 week after symptoms begin. Symptomatic infection depends on age of acquisition. Approximately 10% of children who become infected are symptomatic. In countries of high endemicity, clinical disease is rare, as greater than 90% of people are infected as children and become subsequently immune by adulthood. In countries of lower endemicity, symptomatic infection is seen in adolescents and adults of high-risk groups, such as injection drug users, men having sex with men, travelers to high-prevalence areas, and members of closed religious communities.[1] As a result, HAV presents a significant economic burden to countries of low prevalence, such as the United States.[1]

Early infection is characterized by malaise, fatigue, fever, anorexia, nausea, and abdominal pain, followed by jaundice and dark urine.[2,3] Symptoms usually last no more than 2 months, but can persist or relapse up to 6 months after initial infection in 10% to 15% of patients.[4] Fulminant hepatitis occurs in 0.01% of cases. Liver function rapidly deteriorates, and fatality rates are high when this occurs.

Risk factors

Humans are the only reservoir for HAV. Transmission occurs via the fecal-oral route, person-to-person contact, or contaminated food and water. Much less commonly, cases have been reported after intravenous drug use, blood transfusion, and sexual contact, although usually during the early stages of disease when HAV viral loads are highest.[3] Travel to endemic areas, household contacts of infected persons, and day care and health care settings are all known risk factors, although up to half of patients have no identifiable risk factor.

Prevalence/incidence/mortality rates

The incidence of HAV varies according to the socioeconomic development of the area. Globally approximately 1.4 million new cases of hepatitis A are diagnosed each year.[1] In 2011, the overall incidence rate in the United States was 0.4 per 100,000 population.[5] Since the introduction of the HAV vaccine in 1995, the incidence has decreased by 95% in the United States.[6] Mortality from acute infection is less than 1% but can be higher in the setting of preexisting liver disease.[3,7]

Clinical Outcomes (Pregnancy/Maternal/Fetal)

Acute HAV infection during pregnancy is rare. As a result, incidence during pregnancy is difficult to ascertain. Most cases reported in the literature are those requiring hospitalization and/or recorded in countries endemic for HAV where acute infection in the adult population is low.[2] For example, Elinav and colleagues[2] found that only 13 of 79,458 pregnancies admitted to an Israeli hospital over a 25-year period were diagnosed with acute HAV. During the HAV epidemic in Tennessee from 1994 to 1995, only 4 of the 1700 cases reported were pregnant women.[8]

In general, maternal and fetal outcomes are excellent in developed nations. Preterm birth has been associated with HAV infection in the second and third trimesters, in addition to neonatal cholestasis.[2,9] In the same series from Israel,[2] the average gestational age at delivery in women with HAV was 34 weeks. When fever and hypoalbuminemia (defined as albumin <30 g/L) was present, delivery was significantly earlier, at a mean gestational age of 32 weeks.[2] Hepatitis A is not teratogenic, and transmission to a fetus antepartum, intrapartum, and postpartum via breast milk is rare.

Management

Diagnosis

Diagnosis requires serologic testing. The presence of HAV immunoglobulin M (IgM) is diagnostic of acute infection and persists for several months. HAV IgG predominates during the convalescence stage and provides lifelong immunity. The presence of total anti-HAV antibody indicates past infection but does not differentiate between acute and chronic infection. Anti-HAV IgG is also positive after HAV immunization.[3]

Prevention
Prevention of HAV includes active and passive immunoprophylaxis. The HAV vaccine is available as a single-antigen vaccine or in combination with hepatitis B virus (HBV) vaccine. Both vaccines contain inactivated virus and are safe for use during pregnancy. The single-antigen vaccine is given in 2 doses, 6 to 12 months apart. The combination vaccine is approved for persons 18 years old and upward, and is given in 3 doses at 0-, 1-, and 6-month intervals. After 1 month, 94% to 100% of adults achieve protective levels of IgG and 100% of persons achieve immunity after the second dose. Equivalent immunogenicity is achieved with the combination vaccine. Protective levels of anti-HAV IgG have been shown to persist for 20 years.[3,7]

Immune globulin is also available for postexposure prophylaxis. It is prepared from pooled human plasma and is given as a 0.02 mL/kg dose within 2 weeks of exposure. Vaccination with single-antigen hepatitis A vaccine is, however, the preferred prophylaxis for persons aged 12 to 40 years. If immune globulin is administered, HAV vaccine should still be administered as soon as possible.[3,7] HAV vaccine and immunoglobulin have been shown to be equally effective in preventing HAV if given within 2 weeks of exposure.[10]

Universal vaccination is not recommended.[1,3,7] Instead, vaccination is recommended based on medical or behavioral risk factors. Medical indications for vaccination include persons with chronic liver disease or those receiving clotting factor concentrates. Behavioral indications include illegal drug use, men having sex with men, or travel to areas with medium to high endemicity. Occupational indications for vaccination include working with HAV in a research laboratory setting, including HAV-infected primates. A list of countries where vaccination is recommended before travel is available at http://www.cdc.gov/travel/diseases.htm.[3,7]

Treatment
Management of HAV includes supportive therapy. Outpatient management is undertaken in most cases. Hospitalization is recommended for intractable vomiting, encephalopathy, coagulopathy, or severe debilitation. Nutrition should be maintained and physical activity limited, with the upper abdomen protected from trauma. Close contacts should receive immunoprophylaxis.[3,7] In the rare case of active infection during labor and delivery, appropriate infectious disease precautions should be undertaken with notification of the neonatologist to possible exposure of the infant. Vaginal delivery is not contraindicated. Although HAV RNA has been documented in the breast milk, no cases of vertical transmission have been reported, so breastfeeding is not contraindicated.[11]

Complications and Concerns

As already stated, pregnancy outcomes with HAV are generally good. Fulminant hepatic failure complicates fewer than 1% of acute HAV cases and has been reported during pregnancy. In 2012, Simsek and colleagues[12] reported on a patient at 18 weeks of gestation who presented with acute hepatic failure, encephalopathy, and positive HAV serologies. She underwent a liver transplant with histology positive for acute necrotizing hepatitis A. Although the pregnancy was complicated by severe midtrimester oligohydramnios necessitating termination, she had an otherwise uneventful recovery.

Summary

HAV is an acute, self-limiting infection that does not result in chronic infection. It is endemic in developing countries where greater than 90% of adults have evidence of past infection. By contrast, epidemics can occur in industrialized countries where improved sanitation results in most adults being susceptible. The main route of transmission is fecal-oral spread. Incidence during pregnancy is low, and mortality from fulminant hepatic failure is rare. Preterm birth has been documented after infection in the second and third trimester. Diagnosis is established with serologic testing for HAV IgM and IgG. Routine obstetric management is recommended, and breastfeeding is not contraindicated. HAV vaccine is safe during pregnancy and is recommended based on medical, occupational, and lifestyle risk factors. Postexposure prophylaxis includes immune globulin in addition to HAV vaccination, both of which offer equal protection if given within 2 weeks after exposure.

HEPATITIS B VIRUS
Introduction

Disease description

HBV is a double-stranded DNA virus and a member of the Hepadnaviridae family. This virus preferentially infects liver cells but can also be found in kidney, pancreas, and mononuclear cells, although to a much lesser degree.[13–16] Hepatocellular injury is thought to result from the host immune response to viral antigens and not from DNA replication directly.[17] Hepatitis B can cause both acute and chronic hepatitis.

Risk factors

Transmission occurs via parental or mucosal exposure to infected body fluids. Concentrations are higher in blood and serous fluids than those found in semen and saliva.[18] In low-prevalence countries (prevalence <2%) such as the United States, sexual contact is the major route of transmission. In countries endemic for HBV (prevalence 8%–15%), perinatal exposure accounts for most transmissions.[19,20] As a result, pregnancy poses a particular opportunity to affect the epidemiology of HBV.

Prevalence/incidence/mortality rates

Each year HBV affects 350 million people worldwide. In the United States, an estimated 800,000 to 1.4 million people are living with hepatitis B. Since the implementation of routine childhood vaccination in 1990, the rate of acute hepatitis B in the United States has declined 82%,[20] and in 2011 the national rate of HBV was 0.9 per 100,000 population. The risk of developing chronic hepatitis B is inversely related to age at infection, with 90% of infants, 30% of children younger than 5 years, and only 2% to 6% of those infected as adults progressing to chronic disease.[3] Of those who develop chronic HBV, 15% to 40% will develop severe complications including cirrhosis, liver failure, and hepatocellular carcinoma.[21] As a result, it is estimated that hepatitis B contributes to 786,000 deaths worldwide each year.[22]

Clinical Outcomes (Pregnancy, Maternal, Infant)

The course of HBV in pregnancy is similar to that in the general population. The incubation period ranges from 6 weeks to 6 months (average 75 days), and only 50% of infected persons will be symptomatic.[20,22] Symptomatic disease includes nausea, vomiting, abdominal pain, fatigue, and jaundice. The risk of fulminant hepatic failure and death after acute infection is approximately 1%.[22]

Despite earlier evidence suggesting increased maternal morbidity and mortality, recent evidence from large population-based cohorts suggest that pregnancy is not significantly affected by HBV.[23,24] Reddick and colleagues[24] reviewed 297,664 pregnancies from the Nationwide Inpatient Sample and found a slight increase in preterm birth (adjusted odds ratio 1.65, 95% confidence interval 1.3–2.0) but no association with intrauterine growth restriction or preeclampsia. In 2011 Connell and colleagues[23] reviewed 1,670,369 records and found no increase in adverse pregnancy outcomes in women with HBV, but rather a decreased risk of babies being small for gestational age.

Management

Diagnosis

The diagnosis of HBV is based on laboratory testing. **Fig. 1** illustrates the pattern of the varying HBV antigens and antibodies in acute infection. Hepatitis B surface antigen (HBsAg) and hepatitis e antigen (HBeAg) appear first, followed by IgM antibody to hepatitis B core antigen. This combination of antigens and antibodies is characteristic of acute infection. The presence of IgG anticore or IgG antisurface indicates resolving or past infection. IgG antisurface is also positive in vaccinated persons and is evidence of lifelong immunity.[22] Persistence of HBsAg greater than 6 months signifies chronic infection, and HBeAg indicates ongoing viral replication and infectivity regardless of time from initial infection (**Table 1**). Women positive for HBsAg are considered infected, and should have HBeAg and HBV viral load sent to guide management and counseling. This strategy, in combination with maternal antiviral treatment if positive, has been found to be cost-effective in the prevention of perinatal infection.[25]

The American College of Obstetricians and Gynecologists (ACOG), the Centers for Disease Control and Prevention (CDC), the World Health Organization (WHO), and the US Preventive Services Task Force recommend universal screening of all pregnant

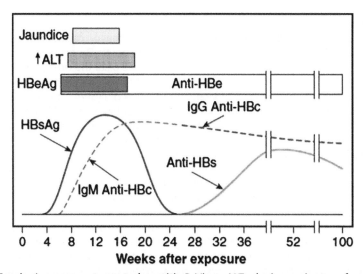

Fig. 1. Serologic response to acute hepatitis B Virus. ALT, alanine aminotransferase; anti-HBc, antibody to hepatitis B core antigen; anti-HBe, antibody to hepatitis B e antigen; anti-HBs, antibody to hepatitis B surface antigen; HBeAg, hepatitis B e antigen; HBsAg, hepatitis B surface antigen; IgG, immunoglobulin G; IgM, immunoglobulin M. (*Adapted from* Dienstag JL. Acute viral hepatitis. In: Longo DL, Fauci AS, Kasper DL, et al, editors. Harrison's principles of internal medicine, 18th edition. New York: McGraw-Hill; 2012. p. 2540.)

Table 1
Interpretation of serologic test results for hepatitis B virus

	Serologic Marker			
HBsAg	Total Anti-HBc	IgM Anti-HBc	Anti-HBs	Interpretation
−	−	−	−	Never infected
+	−	−	−	Early acute infection or first 18 d after vaccination
+	+	+	−	Acute infection
−	+	+	−	Acute infection but resolving
+	+	−	−	Chronic infection
−	+	−	+	Immune from past infection
−	−	−	+	Post HBV vaccination
−	+	−	−	False positive; low-level chronic infection or passive transfer to infant born to HBsAg-positive mother

Abbreviations: Anti-HBc, antibody to hepatitis B core antigen; Anti-HBs, antibody to HBsAg; HBsAg, hepatitis B surface antigen; IgM, immunoglobulin M.

Adapted from Centers for Disease Control and Prevention. Sexually transmitted disease treatment guidelines 2010. MMWR Recomm Rep 2010;59(RR-12):1–110.

women using HBsAg.[3,7,20,26] In a recent retrospective review of all pregnancies infected with HBV from 2007 to 2011 in a single United Kingdom hospital, 71% of mothers were first diagnosed during pregnancy.[27] Thus, pregnancy provides a unique opportunity for screening and identification of HBV in a population that serves as a viral reservoir for future generations.

Treatment

Treatment of acute hepatitis B during pregnancy is mainly supportive. As already stated, vertical transmission is more likely if acute hepatitis B occurs during the third trimester.[28] After acute infection, 85% to 90% of adults clear the virus and the remaining 10% to 15% develop chronic infection. Treatment of chronic hepatitis B outside of pregnancy depends on the level of viremia, presence of HBeAg, and degree of liver injury determined by either transaminase levels or liver histology.[29] Most women during pregnancy are in the immune-tolerant stage (elevated HBV viral load but normal transaminases). However, certain situations arise whereby antiviral treatment is considered. If pregnancy occurs while on treatment, discontinuation of antiviral medication has been associated with rebound hepatitis and liver decompensation.[30] Similarly, antiviral therapy is considered if the woman is newly diagnosed and found to have cirrhosis. However, the main role of antiviral therapy during pregnancy is as prophylaxis against vertical transmission.

Intrapartum management of HBsAg-positive mothers generally does not deviate from routine obstetric management. Although no studies have been performed evaluating the impact of invasive fetal monitoring on vertical transmission rates, it seems reasonable to avoid based on theoretic risks. When preterm premature rupture of membranes (PPROM) complicates antenatal care of seropositive women, pregnancy prolongation can be undertaken, as fetal exposure to HBV-positive maternal fluids and maternal-fetal microtransfusion remain low in the absence of active labor.[31]

It has been hypothesized that elective cesarean delivery might have an advantage over vaginal delivery in terms of vertical transmission rates because fetal exposure to maternal blood and body fluids is minimized before the onset of labor or rupture of membranes. A recent retrospective review from China found that of the 1409 infants born of HBV-seropositive women, vertical transmission occurred only when the maternal viral load exceeded 10^6. Elective cesarean delivery was associated with a lower vertical transmission rate (1.6%) when compared with vaginal delivery (3.6%) or urgent cesarean delivery (4.6%) despite adequate neonatal immunoprophylaxis, leading the investigators to conclude that in mothers with high viral loads, elective cesarean delivery might be associated with lower rates of vertical transmission.[32] By contrast, other studies have found that elective cesarean delivery is not protective. More evidence is needed before a change is made to current recommendations regarding route of delivery.[7]

During the postpartum period, transmission can occur through direct contact with infected household members and, rarely, via breastfeeding.[33] The ACOG and the CDC do not discourage breastfeeding in infants who have received appropriate immunoprophylaxis.[7,28] Exceptions include women receiving antiviral therapy, as limited data are available regarding drug excretion into human breast milk.[34]

Prevention

Prevention of mother-to-child-transmission can occur at both the maternal and neonatal level. The US Food and Drug Administration (FDA) has approved 2 products for prevention of hepatitis B: hepatitis B immune globulin (HBIG), and the hepatitis B vaccine. Routine vaccination is recommended for high-risk populations, which include persons with multiple sex partners, men who have sex with men, intravenous drug users, health care workers, those coinfected with other sexually transmitted diseases, members of correctional facilities and/or drug treatment centers, or those in direct contact with an HBV-positive household member.[3] The hepatitis B vaccine contains recombinant HBsAg prepared from yeast cultures. It is safe in pregnancy and during breastfeeding. Three sequential injections are required for complete serologic protection, traditionally given at an interval of 0, 1, and 6 months. However, this dosing interval may be difficult to complete during pregnancy.[7] Sheffield and colleagues[35] showed that an accelerated dosing schedule at 0, 1, and 4 months resulted in improved rates of completion and a 90% seroconversion rate after 3 doses.

HBIG is composed of plasma from pooled donors with high concentrations of anti-HBs IgG. If used alone for postexposure prophylaxis, protective levels of antibodies last 3 to 6 months.[36,37] Most commonly it is given as an adjunct to the HBV vaccine. In the neonate, passive-active immunoprophylaxis of the infant with HBIG and the hepatitis B vaccine has been shown to be 95% effective for preventing neonatal infection if given within 12 to 24 hours after delivery.[38]

In mothers with high HBV viremia (>10^6 copies per mL), treatment with antiviral medication initiated in the third trimester has been shown to decrease the rate of vertical transmission to the newborn. No consensus exists on which antiviral is best for this indication. Lamivudine, a cytidine nucleoside analogue, is the most studied antiviral during pregnancy given its use in human immunodeficiency virus (HIV) infection, and has a reassuring safety profile. In a systematic review of 10 randomized controlled trials, Shi and colleagues[39] found that initiating lamivudine at 28 to 32 weeks of gestation had a 1.4% to 2.0% lower transmission rate without higher complications rates. Telbivudine is another option in the same drug class with similar efficacy but with less resistance than lamivudine.[40] Tenofovir disoproxil fumarate (TDF) is a class B medication that has also been used for prevention of vertical transmission of HBV. Although data are limited in HBV-positive pregnancies, TDF use in the third trimester has shown a benefit without adverse effects on pregnancy.[41,42] In addition, HBIG given in the third trimester to women with high viremia reduces vertical transmission.[39] Both antiviral therapy and HBIG given to the mother antenatally have been shown to be cost-effective.[43]

Complications and Concerns

Maternal viremia, one of the strongest risk factors for vertical transmission, is measured directly using the level of HBV DNA or indirectly by the presence of HBeAg, a viral protein synthesized in concordance with HBV DNA transcription.[28] Even in the presence of adequate neonatal immunoprophylaxis, there is a 8% to 10% failure rate in HBeAg-positive mothers with high levels of HBV DNA.[41,44] Transmission rates to the neonate are lower in this high-risk group for those women receiving antiviral therapy during the third trimester.[39,41,42]

Vertical transmission can occur antepartum, intrapartum, or postpartum. In acute hepatitis B infection during the first trimester, 10% of infants will become infected, compared with 80% to 90% when acute infection occurs during the third trimester.[28] Amniocentesis is not contraindicated in HBV-positive gravidas. In 1999, Alexander and colleagues[45] found that none of the 21 infants whose mothers were chronic HBV carriers and underwent midtrimester amniocentesis tested positive for HBsAg during the first year of life. By contrast, more contemporary evidence taking into account the level of maternal viremia found that the vertical transmission rate after midtrimester amniocentesis was significantly higher when the maternal viral load exceeded 10^7 copies/mL.[46] Although more evidence is needed to change current recommendations, the level of maternal viremia should be taken into account before proceeding with any invasive antepartum procedure.

Summary

HBV is a double-stranded DNA virus that affects 350 million people worldwide. Transmission occurs via parental or mucosal exposure to infected body fluids. In countries endemic for HBV, perinatal transmission is the major route of infection. All pregnant women should be tested for HBV at least once during pregnancy. Infection is marked by the presence of HBsAg. If positive, HBeAg and HBV DNA level should be obtained for management planning and patient counseling. Risk of perinatal infection without infant immunoprophylaxis is 10% and rises to 80% when HBeAg is present. Level of maternal viremia also influences vertical transmission rates, with viral loads greater than 10^6 associated with higher rates of perinatal infections. It is unclear if elective cesarean delivery reduces vertical transmission rates. Breastfeeding is not contraindicated. Treatment of HBV during pregnancy is mainly supportive. HBV vaccine is recommended for high-risk groups and can be administered at 0, 1, and 6 months or via an accelerated schedule of 0, 1, and 4 months with equal efficacy. All infants born to HBV-positive mothers should receive HBIG and HBV vaccine within 24 hours of birth. Maternal antiviral therapy starting at 28 to 32 weeks has been shown to reduce rates of perinatal infection without adverse effects.

HEPATITIS C
Introduction

Disease description
Hepatitis C is the most common blood-borne infection in the United States. Hepatitis C virus (HCV) is an RNA virus from the Flaviviridae family[47] and possesses an error-prone RNA replicase, which is responsible for the genetic heterogeneity between the 6 major HCV genotypes. Genetic diversity of HCV has complicated antiviral

therapy and is one of the main reasons why seroconversion does not provide lifelong immunity.[48] Genotype 1 accounts for most infections in the United States.

Risk factors

Hepatitis C is a blood-borne infection, and transmission most commonly occurs through exchange of infected blood and body fluids. Populations at highest risk include intravenous drug users (IVDU) and those receiving infected blood products.[49] It is estimated that 60% to 80% of IVDU are infected with hepatitis C. Since screening of blood products began in 1992, the risk of acquiring HCV after a blood transfusion is now estimated to be 1 in 2 million transfusions.[50] Transmission less commonly occurs perinatally or through sexual contact.[3] Both HIV coinfection and numerous sexual partners increases the likelihood of sexual transmission.[3]

Prevalence/incidence/mortality rates

It is estimated that greater than 4.8 million people are chronically infected in North America, a prevalence rate of 1.3%.[49] The incidence of HCV during pregnancy is 1% to 2.4%.[7] Of infants born to seropositive women, 6 in 100 will acquire HCV perinatally,[50,51] translating into almost 2500 perinatally acquired infections annually.

Clinical Outcomes (Pregnancy, Maternal, Fetal)

Most HCV infections are asymptomatic and are discovered either from screening high-risk groups or during evaluation of persistent transaminitis. Symptoms of abdominal pain, nausea, vomiting, and fatigue can develop 1 to 3 months after infection. Jaundice occurs in 10% to 15% of acute infections, and has been shown to correlate with clearance of acute infection.[48] Severe acute disease leading to hepatic failure is rare. Up to 85% of patients develop chronic HCV. Progression to cirrhosis is related to the patient's age at initial infection in addition to alcohol consumption and degree of immunosuppression.[52-54] HCV RNA can be detected in blood 1 to 3 weeks after initial infection, and seroconversion occurs by 6 months.[3]

Most HCV infected pregnant women have chronic disease. It was previously thought that HCV had limited effects on pregnancy. However, recent reports have shown an association with intrahepatic cholestasis of pregnancy, gestational diabetes, and preterm delivery in seropositive gravidas.[23,24,55,56] Adverse fetal outcomes reported include an increased incidence of congenital anomalies, low birth weight, newborns small for gestational age, need for assisted ventilation, and requirement of neonatal intensive care.[23] Most recent data suggest that HCV seropositivity during pregnancy is associated with an adverse neurologic outcome, cephalohematoma, fetal distress, feeding difficulties, intraventricular hemorrhage, and neonatal seizure.[57]

Management

Diagnosis

Routine prenatal screening is not recommended. The CDC and the ACOG recommend risk-based testing during pregnancy to include women with past or current intravenous drug use, HIV positivity, history of blood transfusion and/or solid organ transplant before 1992, history of having received clotting factor concentrates before 1987, undergoing long-term dialysis, signs/symptoms of liver disease, and seeking treatment at STD clinics.[3,7] Antibody to HCV, using either a second-generation or third-generation enzyme immunoassay, is used for screening. Seroconversion may not be evident for 6 to 10 weeks after acute infection; therefore if anti-HCV is negative but clinical suspicion remains high, HCV RNA using polymerase chain reaction can be detected soon after initial infection.[7]

Most patients during pregnancy who test positive for antibody to HCV have chronic disease. Quantification of HCV RNA is useful for patient counseling, as high levels of maternal viremia have been associated with higher rates of vertical transmission.[58] Although human leukocyte antigen variations and mismatches between the mother and her infant have been shown to be prognostic in terms of vertical transmission rates,[59] genetic testing is currently not recommended. Full evaluation of liver function, presence of cirrhosis, and presence of other organ system dysfunction is warranted for both staging and prognosis. Liver biopsy is usually deferred until after delivery.

Prevention

Unlike HBV, no vaccine or immunoprophylaxis is available for HCV-positive women or their neonates. Rates of transmission have been shown to be as low as 0% to 3% when maternal HCV RNA was undetectable.[51,58,60] Women who are HCV negative but remain at high risk of acquisition should be educated regarding practices that decrease the risk of transmission.[3] Because the risk of sexual transmission is low, serodiscordant monogamous couples do not need to change their sexual practices, but should be tested regularly.[3] HCV disease is not a contraindication to breastfeeding.

Treatment

The preferred treatment of chronic HCV is a combination of pegylated interferon and ribavirin, both of which are contraindicated during pregnancy. Ribavirin has been shown to be teratogenic and pegylated interferon has been shown to have adverse effects on fetal growth.[61] Newer treatment options include direct-acting antivirals, which target specific steps in the HCV viral replication cycle. These agents have less morbidity than nonspecific therapy, and shorter treatment times.[49,62,63] However, their safety during pregnancy has not been established, and studies are needed before recommending treatment with these antivirals. Seropositive women with systemic complications from HCV should be comanaged by both maternal-fetal medicine specialists and gastroenterologists specializing in viral hepatitis.

The mode of delivery has not been shown to affect vertical transmission rates for HCV-positive women.[51,64] Invasive procedures, such as fetal scalp electrode or fetal scalp sampling, should be avoided, as these procedures have been shown to increase vertical transmission rates.[58] Evidence is lacking regarding the risk of transmission after amniocentesis, although no evidence suggests an increased risk.[65] If amniocentesis is performed, traversing the placenta should be avoided. Vertical transmission has been shown to be higher after premature rupture of membranes. However, this could be related to maternal viral load and length of membrane rupture. Recent data from Japan noted that in women with high viral loads (defined as $>6 \times 10^5$ IU/mL), delivery 4 or more hours after membrane rupture was associated with a significantly higher rate of infected infants.[66] Further studies are needed before recommendations can be made as regards management of PPROM in seropositive pregnancies. Breastfeeding does not seem to increase transmission rates, and is therefore not contraindicated unless the nipples are cracked and/or bleeding.[3,67]

Complications and Concerns

Vertical transmission can occur at any time during gestation. One-third of transmissions occur antepartum, 40% to 50% occur peripartum, and transmission during the postpartum period is rare.[68] Risk appears to be greatest in women with an

RNA viral load greater than 2.5×10^6 RNA copies/mL[58] and those with HIV coinfection. Vertical transmission can be as high as 15% to 25% in women with coincident HIV.[58] Although highly active antiretroviral therapy reduces HIV transmission to the neonate, it remains unclear whether HCV vertical transmission is similarly affected.[69]

Summary

HCV is the most common blood-borne infection in the United States. Approximately 1.2 million people, including 1% to 2.4% of pregnant women, are chronically infected. Risk factors include intravenous drug use and blood/body fluid contact. Most acute infections are asymptomatic, and 85% of infected patients develop chronic disease with the potential for cirrhosis and hepatocellular carcinoma. Retrospective reviews have reported an increase in preterm birth, low birth weight, neonates small for gestational age, requirement of neonatal intensive care, congenital anomalies, and adverse neurologic outcomes in HCV-positive mothers, although outcomes are generally favorable. There is no vaccine for HCV. Testing during pregnancy is recommended for high-risk patients. Treatment during pregnancy is supportive, and invasive procedures should be avoided. Perinatal transmission is not influenced by mode of delivery, but does appear to be increased with high maternal viremia and HIV coinfection. Breastfeeding is not contraindicated. HCV-positive women should have long-term follow-up conducted by a hepatologist.

HEPATITIS D
Introduction

Disease description
Hepatitis D virus (HDV) is a small, incomplete RNA virus that requires the HBsAg coat for both transmission and replication. Therefore, monoinfection with HDV does not occur.[70] Coinfection with HBV is associated with more severe acute hepatitis. Progression to cirrhosis occurs in 70% to 80% of patients with chronic disease. In 15%, progression occurs within 2 years.[7,71,72] Similarly to HBV, transmission of HDV occurs through contact with infected blood/body fluids or blood products.[72]

Risk factors
Risk factors for acquiring HDV are similar to those specific to HBV (see earlier discussion in the hepatitis B section under Risk Factors). Patients not immunized against HBV are also susceptible to HDV coinfection.[72]

Incidence/prevalence/mortality rates
It is estimated that 15 million of the 350 million individuals with chronic HBV have also been exposed to HDV.[70] Areas endemic for HBV have the highest rates of HDV infection.[73] Mortality rates after HDV/HBV coinfection are 10 times higher than those for HBV monoinfection.[72] The true incidence of HDV during pregnancy is unknown, as estimates quoted in the literature originate from countries where HBV is endemic.[74–76] In a recent study from Africa, 14.7% of HBV-positive gravidas were coinfected with HDV.[74]

Clinical Outcomes (Pregnancy, Maternal, Infant)

Pregnancy outcomes specific to women with HBV/HDV coinfection have not been reported. Although HBV DNA levels are lower in coinfected women, no evidence exists to suggest better maternal or fetal outcomes.[74]

Management

Diagnosis

The WHO recommends that all women who are HBsAg positive or have evidence of recent HBV infection[72] be tested for HDV. The preferred method of diagnosis is detection of total anti-HDV antibodies. Presence of hepatitis D antigen and HDV RNA is evidence of active liver disease.[71,72] No cases of HDV reinfection have been reported.[72]

Prevention

There is no HDV-specific vaccine. Because HDV requires the presence of HBV for survival, all measures that prevent HBV will also prevent HDV (see section on hepatitis B).

Treatment

Treatment of HBV/HDV coinfection during pregnancy is supportive. Long-term pegylated interferon therapy has yielded remissions, but is contraindicated during pregnancy. Because HDV lacks its own viral polymerase, oral nucleos(t)ides seem to have little effect on HDV viral replication, and addition of these agents is indicated solely for the treatment of HBV.[71–73] In the cases of fulminant hepatic failure and end-stage liver disease, liver transplantation can be life-saving.

Complications and concerns

As already stated, coinfection with HDV causes more severe liver disease with faster progression to cirrhosis and higher mortality rates in comparison with HBV monoinfection.[73] However, rates of hepatocellular carcinoma are not higher with coinfection, perhaps because of HDV suppression of HBV replication.[77]

Summary

HDV is an incomplete RNA virus that requires HBV for transmission and replication. Approximately 15 million people with chronic HBV have evidence of exposure, mainly in areas endemic for HBV. Liver disease is more severe and mortality rates are higher in comparison with HBV monoinfection. Preventive measures against HBV also prevent HDV coinfection. There is no HDV-specific vaccine, and treatment during pregnancy is supportive. Since the adoption of HBV immunoprophylaxis, perinatal transmission of HDV has been rare.

HEPATITIS E
Introduction

Disease description

Hepatitis E virus (HEV) is a single-stranded, nonenveloped RNA virus that has historically been a disease of developing countries, similar to HAV. In recent years, an increasing number of cases have emerged in more developed countries as a result of zoonotic infections from infected, undercooked meats.[78,79] There are 4 genotypes known to infect humans. Genotypes 1 and 2 are endemic in Asia, Africa, Central America, and other developing countries where sanitation is poor. Humans are the only known reservoir, and fecal-oral transmission occurs through water contamination. Genotypes 3 and 4 are more prevalent in developed countries, such as the United States, the United Kingdom, and Japan. These genotypes infect humans and animals, with swine being the main reservoir. Zoonotic spread via consumption of raw or undercooked meat, namely pork or game, has been shown to be the main route of transmission in these countries.

Most HEV infections are asymptomatic. The incubation period ranges from 2 to 8 weeks and symptoms include myalgia, arthralgia, weakness, vomiting, jaundice, itching, acolic stools, and dark urine. The symptomatic phase is accompanied by elevated transaminases and jaundice.[78,80,81] Most infections are self-limiting, but chronic infection can develop in immunocompromised patients.[82] When this occurs, progression to cirrhosis is rapid and can occur 2 to 3 years after infection.[71] One of the features of HEV that most distinguish it from the other hepatides is its particularly virulent course during pregnancy whereby mortality rates from fulminant hepatic failure are estimated to be 10- to 25-fold higher[83,84]; this is seen more frequently with gentoypes 1 and 2. Extrahepatic manifestations of HEV include neurologic symptoms in 2% to 5% of cases, in addition to glomerulonephritis or cryoglobulinemia.[85,86]

Risk factors

In endemic areas where sanitation is poor, HEV is acquired through contaminated drinking water. In industrialized countries where genotypes 3 and 4 predominate, infection mainly occurs from ingestion of infected meats, mainly pork or deer meat. Feagins and colleagues[87] found that 11% of pig livers obtained from grocery stores in the United States contained HEV RNA. Cooking temperature greater than 70°C for 20 minutes is necessary to inactivate the virus. Persons who have direct contact with infected animals, such as pig handlers and/or veterinarians, are also at risk of infection through infected water. Transmission can also occur through blood transfusions and solid organ donations. Perinatal transmission of HEV during acute infection has been documented,[88] and the risk of transmission can be as high as 79%.[89] However, this estimate is limited by small case series, limited surveillance, and underdiagnosis of HEV during pregnancy.

Prevalence/incidence/mortality rates

The prevalence of HEV IgG antibody is as high as 50% in endemic countries. Globally there are an estimated 20 million cases of HEV reported each year, and more than 3 million are symptomatic. The overall mortality rate is less than 1%, with approximately 57,000 to 70,000 deaths each year.[81,90] As HEV can be particularly virulent during pregnancy, most deaths reported are in pregnant women. The WHO estimates that the risk of death in the third trimester is 20%.[81]

Clinical Outcomes (Pregnancy, Maternal, Infant)

Most studies performed on HEV-infected pregnant populations were conducted in countries of high endemicity. From these populations, where genotypes 1 and 2 predominate, pregnancy outcomes differ depending on severity of infection. High rates of preterm delivery and perinatal mortality have been reported.[91,92] A recent prospective study of 36 HEV-positive pregnant women in India found significantly higher rates of encephalopathy (30.5%), coagulopathy (72.2%), and intrauterine demise (55.5%) when compared with HBV-positive pregnancies. Further, all maternal deaths (n = 5) occurred in HEV-positive women.[93] Gravidas who experience acute liver failure have worse pregnancy outcomes than those who have only acute hepatitis. Borkakoti and colleagues[94] found a 56% death rate in pregnant women with acute hepatic failure, compared with 0.9% in those with acute HEV hepatitis. Gravidas with acute HEV liver failure also had significantly higher rates of intrauterine death (78.6% vs 11.4%), preterm delivery (65.7% vs 17.3%), and maternal mortality (56.2% vs 0.9%). The question as to why HEV has such a virulent course during pregnancy remains to be answered. Elevated levels of tumor necrosis factor α and cytokine gene polymorphisms have been found in HEV-positive pregnant women in comparison with nonpregnant populations.[95,96] Viral load seems to play a factor, at least indirectly. Women with HEV during pregnancy have higher viral loads that are proportional to disease severity.[92,94] Studies of pregnancy outcomes in industrialized, nonendemic countries are lacking. In a recent study from France, HEV seroprevalence during pregnancy was unexpectedly high (29.3%) in contrast to the lack of symptomatic disease, suggesting that most infection during pregnancy was subclinical or asymptomatic.[97]

Vertical transmission of HEV has been reported, and can occur at any point during pregnancy. Reported transmission rates are as high as 67% in women with symptomatic infection.[88] Unlike HBV or HCV, HEV is often self-limited in the neonate. Progression to fulminant hepatitis is rare.[88] No studies have evaluated whether HEV can be transmitted through breastfeeding, so recommendations are lacking.[88]

Management

Diagnosis

It is difficult to distinguish HEV from other forms of acute hepatitis, so a high degree of suspicion is warranted. Testing is indicated in any patient with unexplained hepatitis regardless of age or travel history.[81] Diagnostic markers of infection include HEV RNA, HEV IgM, and HEV IgG. If HEV IgM or IgG are positive, confirmatory testing with HEV RNA should be ordered. Serology can be falsely negative in immunocompromised patients; therefore, HEV RNA testing is recommended if clinically suspected in this population.[71] Persistently positive HEV RNA and rising IgG titers are characteristic of chronic infection.[71,84] HEV IgG does not confer protective immunity.[84]

Prevention

There is no FDA-approved vaccine against HEV.[81] However, 2 different recombinant vaccines have been developed that show high efficacy against HEV.[83] Though promising, more data are needed in pregnant populations before widespread immunization is recommended. Other preventive measures include avoiding use or consumption of water of unknown purity, especially in areas endemic for HEV. Such measures include use of bottled water and avoidance of food cleaned with local water.[81] In countries where genotypes 3 and 4 predominate, meats should be cooked at temperatures higher than 70°C for at least 20 minutes to inactivate the virus.[84]

Treatment

Treatment of HEV during pregnancy is supportive. Ribavirin (and in some instances pegylated interferon) has been used in nonpregnant populations to assist viral clearance, but is contraindicated during pregnancy.[84] The main treatment of HEV is through prevention (see earlier discussion).

Complications and Concerns

Hepatitis E causes a disproportionate number of deaths during pregnancy from acute liver failure in developing countries. Prevention can be achieved through good hygiene practices and improved sanitation, and clinical trials of vaccine efficacy are promising.

Summary

HEV is the most common cause of acute hepatitis worldwide. Genotypes 1 and 2 are common in developing countries where sanitation and water purity is poor, making fecal-oral transmission the main route of acquisition. Acute viral hepatitis with fulminant hepatic failure and death are distinguishing features during pregnancy, with a 20% risk of maternal mortality during the third trimester. Other adverse pregnancy outcomes include preterm delivery, intrauterine death, and vertical transmission. Genotypes 3 and 4 predominate in industrialized countries, and the main route of transmission is through undercooked meats from infected animals, mainly pork. The disease course of HEV during pregnancy is much less virulent. HEV is usually self-limited, but can become chronic in immunocompromised patients. Diagnosis is made by identification of HEV IgM and/or IgG and is confirmed by the presence of HEV RNA. Treatment is supportive. Although no vaccines have been approved for use in the United States, there are 2 vaccines currently available to at-risk populations in China. Further studies of pregnant patients are needed before universal vaccination is recommended.

REFERENCES

HEPATITIS A

1. World Health Organization. Available at: http://www.who.int/mediacentre/factsheets/fs328/en/. Accessed April 28, 2014.
2. Elinav E, Ben-Dov IZ, Shapira Y, et al. Acute hepatitis A infection in pregnancy is associated with high rates of gestational complications and preterm labor. Gastroenterology 2006;130:1129–34.
3. Centers for Disease Control. Sexually transmitted disease treatment guidelines 2010. MMWR Recomm Rep 2010;59(RR-12):1–110.
4. Dienstag JL. Acute viral hepatitis. In: Longo DL, Fauci AS, Kasper DL, et al, editors. Harrison's principles of internal medicine. 18th edition. New York: McGraw-Hill; 2012. p. 2537–57.
5. Centers for Disease Control and Prevention. Division of Viral Hepatitis. Viral hepatitis statistics and surveillance – surveillance for viral hepatitis, United States 2011. Available at: http://www.cdc.gov/hepatitis/Statistics/2011Surveillance/Commentary.htm#hepA. Accessed April 28, 2014.
6. Centers for Disease Control and Prevention. Hepatitis A information for health professionals. Available at: http://www.cdc.gov/hepatitis/HAV/HAVfaq.htm#general. Accessed May 23, 2014.
7. American College of Obstetricians and Gynecologists. ACOG Practice Bulletin No. 86: Viral hepatitis in pregnancy. Obstet Gynecol 2007;110:941–55 Reaffirmed 2012.
8. Willner IR, Howard SC, Williams EQ, et al. Serious hepatitis A: an analysis of patients hospitalized during an urban epidemic in the United States. Ann Intern Med 1998;128:111–4.
9. Urganci N, Arapoglu M, Akyildiz B, et al. Neonatal cholestasis resulting from vertical transmission of hepatitis A infection. Pediatr Infect Dis J 2003;22(4):381–2.
10. Victor JC, Monto AS, Surdina TY, et al. Hepatitis A vaccine versus immune globulin for postexposure prophylaxis. N Engl J Med 2007;357(7):1685–94.
11. Daudi N, Shouval D, Stein-Zamir C, et al. Breastmilk hepatitis A virus RNA in nursing mothers with acute hepatitis A virus infection. Breastfeed Med 2012;7:313–5.
12. Simsek Y, Isik B, Karaer A, et al. Fulminant hepatitis A infection in second trimester of pregnancy requiring living-donor liver transplantation. J Obstet Gynaecol Res 2012;38(4):745–8.

HEPATITIS B

13. Marion PL. Use of animal models to study hepatitis B viruses. Prog Med Virol 1988;35:43–75.

14. Korba BE, Gowans EJ, Well FV, et al. Systemic distribution of woodchuck hepatitis virus in the tissues of experimentally infected woodchucks. Virology 1988; 165:172–81.

15. Halpern MS, England JM, Deery JT, et al. Viral nucleic acid synthesis and antigen accumulation in pancreas and kidney of Peking ducks infected with duck hepatitis B virus. Proc Natl Acad Sci U S A 1983;80:4865–9.

16. Barker LF, Maynard JE, Purcell RH, et al. Hepatitis B virus infection in chimpanzees: titration of subtypes. J Infect Dis 1975;132:451–8.

17. Stevens CE, Beasley RP, Tsui J, et al. Vertical transmission of hepatitis B antigen in Taiwan. N Engl J Med 1975;292:771–4.

18. Dienstag JL. Hepatitis B virus infection. N Engl J Med 2008;359:1486–500.

19. Kowdley KV, Wang CC, Welch S, et al. Prevalence of chronic hepatitis B among foreign born persons living in the United States by country of origin. Hepatology 2012;56:422–33.

20. World Health Organization. Media Centre. Hepatitis B. Fact sheet. Updated July 2013. Available at: http://www.who.int/mediacentre/factsheets/fs204/en/. Accessed April 4, 2014.

21. Bosch FX, Ribes J, Cleries R, et al. Epidemiology of hepatocellular carcinoma. Clin Liver Dis 2005;9(2):191–211.

22. Centers for Disease Control and Prevention. Hepatitis B information for health professionals. Available at: http://www.cdc.gov/hepatitis/HBV/index.htm. Accessed April 4, 2014.

23. Connell LE, Salihu HM, Salemi JL, et al. Maternal hepatitis B and hepatitis C carrier status and perinatal outcomes. Liver Int 2011;31(8):1163–70.

24. Reddick KLB, Jhaveri R, Gandhi M, et al. Pregnancy outcomes associated with viral hepatitis. J Viral Hepat 2011;18:394–8.

25. Fan L, Owusu-Edusei K, Schillie S, et al. Cost-effectiveness of testing hepatitis B-positive pregnant women for hepatitis B e antigen or viral load. Obstet Gynecol 2014;123:929–37.

26. U.S. Preventive Services Task Force. Screening for hepatitis B infection in pregnancy, topic page. e2009. Available at: http://www.uspreventiveservicestaskforce.org/uspstf/uspshepbpg.htm. Accessed April 27, 2014.

27. Dyson JK, Waller J, Turley A, et al. Hepatitis B in pregnancy. Frontline Gastroenterol 2014;5(2):111–7.

28. Mast EE, Margolis HS, Fiore AE, et al. A comprehensive immunization strategy to eliminate transmission of hepatitis B virus infection in the United States: recommendations of the Advisory Committee on Immunization Practices (ACIP) part 1: immunization of infants, children, and adolescents. Advisory Committee on Immunization Practices (ACIP). MMWR Recomm Rep 2005; 54(RR-16):1–31 [Erratum appears in MMWR Morb Mortal Wkly Rep 2006;55: 158–9].

29. Lok AS, McMahon BJ. Chronic hepatitis B: update 2009. AASLD Practice Guideline Update. Hepatology 2009;50(3):1–36.

30. Patton H, Tran TT. Management of hepatitis B during pregnancy. Nat Rev Gastroenterol Hepatol 2014. http://dx.doi.org/10.1038/nrgastro.2014.30.

31. Lin HH, Lee TY, Chen DS, et al. Transplacental leakage of HBeAg-positive maternal blood as the most likely route in causing intrauterine infection with hepatitis B virus. J Pediatr 1987;111:877–81.

32. Pan CQ, Zou HB, Chen Y, et al. Cesarean section reduces perinatal transmission of hepatitis B virus infection from hepatitis B surface antigen-positive women to their infants. Clin Gastroenterol Hepatol 2013;11:1349–55.

33. Wong VC, Lee AK, Ip HM. Transmission of hepatitis B antigens from symptom free carrier mothers to the fetus and the infant. Br J Obstet Gynaecol 1980;87:958–65.
34. Mirochnik M, Thomas T, Capparelli E, et al. Antiretroviral concentrations in breast-feeding infants of mothers receiving highly active antiretroviral therapy. Antimicrob Agents Chemother 2009;53:1170–6.
35. Sheffield JS, Hickman A, Tang J, et al. Efficacy of an accelerated hepatitis B vaccination program during pregnancy. Obstet Gynecol 2011;117(5):1130–5.
36. Centers for Disease Control and Prevention. A comprehensive immunization strategy to eliminate transmission of hepatitis B virus infection in the United States: recommendations of the Advisory Committee on Immunization Practices (ACIP) Part II: immunization of adults. MMWR Recomm Rep 2006;55(RR-16):1–33.
37. Centers for Disease Control and Prevention. A comprehensive immunization strategy to eliminate transmission of hepatitis B virus infection in the United States: recommendations of the Advisory Committee on Immunization Practices (ACIP) Part 1: immunization of infants, children, and adolescents. MMWR Recomm Rep 2005;54(RR-16):1–33.
38. United States Department of Health and Human Services. MMWR: a comprehensive immunization strategy to eliminate transmission of hepatitis B virus infection in the United States (online). Available at: http://www.cdc.gov/mmwr/preview/mmwrhtml/rr5416a1.htm. Accessed May 10, 2014.
39. Shi Z, Yang Y, Ma L, et al. Lamivudine in late pregnancy to interrupt in utero transmission of hepatitis B virus: A systematic review and meta-analysis. Obstet Gynecol 2010;116(1):147–58 (Systematic review and/or Meta-analysis).
40. Deng M, Zhou X, Gao S, et al. The effects of telbivudine in late pregnancy to prevent intrauterine transmission of the hepatitis B virus: a systematic review and meta-analysis. Virol J 2012;9:185 (Systematic review and/or Meta-analysis).
41. Pan CQ, Duan ZP, Bhamidimarri KR, et al. An algorithm for risk assessment and intervention of mother to child transmission of hepatitis B virus. Clin Gastroenterol Hepatol 2012;10:452–9.
42. Greenup AJ, Tan PK, Nguyen V, et al. Efficacy and safety of tenofovir disoproxil fumarate in pregnancy to prevent perinatal transmission of Hepatitis B virus. J Hepatol 2014. http://dx.doi.org/10.1016/j.jhep.2014.04.038. pii:S0168-8278(14)00301-8.
43. Nayeri UA, Werner EF, Han CS, et al. Antenatal lamivudine to reduce perinatal hepatitis B transmission: a cost-effectiveness analysis. Am J Obstet Gynecol 2012;207:231.e1–7.
44. Zou H, Chen Y, Duan Z, et al. Virologic factors associated with failure to passive-active immunoprophylaxis in infants born to HBsAg-positive mothers. J Viral Hepat 2012;19:e18–25.
45. Alexander JM, Ramus R, Jackson G, et al. Risk of hepatitis B transmission after amniocentesis if chronic hepatitis B carriers. Infect Dis Obstet Gynecol 1999;7(6):283–6.
46. Yi W, Pan CQ, Hao J, et al. Risk of vertical transmission of hepatitis B after amniocentesis in HBs antigen-positive mothers. J Hepatol 2014;60:523–9.

HEPATITIS C

47. Lemons SM, Walker CM. Hepatitis C virus. In: Knipe DM, Howley PM, editors. Fields virology. 5th edition. Philadelphia: Lippincott Williams & Wilkins; 2007. p. 91.
48. Rehermann B, Nascimbeni M. Immunology of hepatitis B virus and hepatitis C virus infection. Nat Rev Immunol 2005;5(3):215–29.

49. World Health Organization. Guidelines for the screening, care and treatment of persons with hepatitis C infection. 2014. Available at: http://apps.who.int/iris/bitstream/10665/111747/1/9789241548755_eng.pdf?ua=1. Accessed May 20, 2014.
50. Centers for Disease Control and Prevention. Hepatitis C information for health professionals. Available at: http://www.cdc.gov/hepatitis/HCV/Index.htm. Accessed May 20, 2014.
51. McMenamin MB, Jackson A, Lambert J, et al. Obstetric management of hepatitis C-positive mothers: analysis of vertical transmission in 559 mother-infant pairs. Am J Obstet Gynecol 2008;199:315.e5.
52. Poynard T, Bedossa P, Opolon P. Natural history of liver fibrosis progression in patients with chronic hepatitis C. The OBSVIRC, METAVIR, CLINIVIR, and DOSVIRC groups. Lancet 1997;349(9055):825–32.
53. Machicao VI, Bonatti H, Krishna M, et al. Donor age affects fibrosis progression and graft survival after liver transplantation for hepatitis C. Transplantation 2004; 77(1):84–92.
54. Thein HH, Yi Q, Dore GJ, et al. Estimation of stage-specific fibrosis progression rates in chronic hepatitis C virus infection: a meta-analysis and meta-regression. Hepatology 2008;48(2):418–31 (Systematic review and/or Meta-analysis).
55. Berkely EM, Leslie KK, Arora S, et al. Chronic hepatitis C in pregnancy. Obstet Gynecol 2008;112(2 part 1):304–10.
56. Pergram SA, Wang CC, Gardella CM, et al. Pregnancy complications associated with hepatitis C: data from a 2003-2005 Washington state birth cohort. Am J Obstet Gynecol 2008;199:38.e1–9.
57. Salemi JL, Whiteman VE, August EM, et al. Maternal hepatitis B and hepatitis C infection and neonatal neurological outcomes. J Viral Hepat 2014. http://dx.doi.org/10.1111/jvh.12250.
58. Mast EE, Hwang LY, Seto DS, et al. Risk factors for perinatal transmission of hepatitis C virus (HCV) and the natural history of HCV infection acquired in infancy. J Infect Dis 2005;192:1880–9.
59. Bevilacqua A, Fabris A, Floreano P, et al. Genetic factors in mother-to-child transmission of HCV infection. Virology 2009;390:64–70.
60. Airoldi J, Berghella V. Hepatitis C and pregnancy. Obstet Gynecol Surv 2006; 61(10):666–72.
61. Chutaputti A. Adverse effects and other safety aspects of the hepatitis C antivirals. J Gastroenterol Hepatol 2000;15:E156–63.
62. De Clercq E. The design of drugs for HIV and HCV. Nat Rev Drug Discov 2007; 6(12):1001–18.
63. Schlutter J. Therapeutics: new drugs hit the target. Nature 2011;474(7350):S5–7.
64. Ghamar Chehreh ME, Tabatabaei SV, Khazanehdari S, et al. Effect of cesarean section on the risk of perinatal transmission of hepatitis C virus from HCV-RNA+/HIV mothers: a meta-analysis. Arch Gynecol Obstet 2011;283:255–60.
65. Lopez M, Coll O. Chronic viral infections and invasive procedures: risk of vertical transmission and current recommendations. Fetal Diagn Ther 2010;28:1–8.
66. Murakami J, Nagata I, Iitsuka T, et al. Risk factors for mother-to-child transmission of hepatitis C virus: Maternal high viral load and fetal exposure in the birth canal. Hepatol Res 2012;42:648–57.
67. Cottrell EB, Chou R, Wasson N, et al. Reducing risk for mother-to-infant transmission of hepatitis C virus: a systematic review for the U.S. Preventive Services Task Force. Ann Intern Med 2013;158:109–13 (Systematic review and/or Meta-analysis).

68. Mok J, Pembrey L, Tovo PA, et al. When does mother to child transmission of hepatitis C virus occur? Arch Dis Child Fetal Neonatal Ed 2005;90:F156–60.
69. European Paediatric Hepatitis C Virus Network. A significant sex-but not elective cesarean section-effect on mother-to-child transmission of hepatitis C virus infection. J Infect Dis 2005;192:1872–9.

HEPATITIS D

70. Centers for Disease Control and Prevention. Division of Viral Hepatitis. Hepatitis D information for health professionals. Available at: www.cdc.gov/hepatitis/HDV/. Accessed May 5, 14.
71. Price J. An update on hepatitis B, D and E viruses. Top Antivir Med 2014;21(5):157–63.
72. World Health Organization. Global alert and response. Hepatitis D virus. Available at: http://www.who.int/csr/disease/hepatitis/whocdscsrncs2001l/en/index3.html. Accessed May 14, 2014.
73. Hughes SA, Wedemeyer H, Harrison PM. Hepatitis delta virus. Lancet 2011; 378(9785):73–85.
74. Mansour W, Malick FZ, Sidiya A, et al. Prevalence, risk factors, and molecular epidemiology of hepatitis B and hepatitis delta virus in pregnancy women and in patients in Mauritania. J Med Virol 2012;84(8):1186–98.
75. Makuwa M, Caron M, Souqiuere S, et al. Prevalence and genetic diversity of hepatitis B and delta viruses in pregnant women in Gabon: molecular evidence that hepatitis delta virus clade 8 originates from and is endemic in central Africa. J Clin Microbiol 2008;46(2):754–6.
76. Drobeniuc J, Hutin YJ, Harpaz R, et al. Prevalence of hepatitis B, C, and D virus infections among children and pregnant women in Moldova: additional evidence supporting the need for routine hepatitis B vaccination of infants. Epidemiol Infect 1999;123:463–7.
77. Cross TJ, Rizzi P, Horner M, et al. The increasing prevalence of hepatitis delta virus (HDV) infection in South London. J Med Virol 2008;80:277–82.

HEPATITIS E

78. Wedemeyer J, Pischke S, Manns M. Pathogenesis and treatment of hepatitis E virus infection. Gastroenterology 2012;142:1388–97.
79. Purcell RH, Emerson SU. Hepatitis E: emerging awareness of an old disease. J Hepatol 2008;48:494–503.
80. Centers for Disease Control and Prevention. Division of viral hepatitis. Hepatitis E information for health professionals. Available at: http://www.cdc.gov/hepatitis/HEV/index.htm. Accessed May 14, 2014.
81. World Health Organization. Hepatitis E fact sheet, updated July 2013. Available at: http://www.who.int/mediacentre/factsheets/fs280/en/. Accessed May 24, 2014.
82. Niet de A, Zaaijer HL, Ten Berge I, et al. Chronic hepatitis E after solid organ transplantation. Neth J Med 2012;70:261–6.
83. Labrique AB, Sikder SS, Krain LJ, et al. Hepatitis e, a vaccine-preventable cause of maternal deaths. Emerg Infect Dis 2012;18(9):1401–4.
84. Scobie L, Dalton HR. Review. Hepatitis E: source and route of infection, clinical manifestations and new developments. J Viral Hepat 2013;20:1–11.
85. Kamar N, Bendall RP, Peron JM, et al. Hepatitis E virus-induced neurologic disorders. Emerg Infect Dis 2011;17:173–9.
86. Kamar N, Weclawski H, Guibeau-Frugier C, et al. Hepatitis E virus and the kidney in solid-organ transplant patients. Transplantation 2012;93(6):617–23.

87. Feagins AR, Opriessing R, Guenette DK, et al. Detection and characterization of infectious Hepatitis E virus from commercial pig livers sold in local grocery stores in the USA. J Gen Virol 2007;88(Pt 3):912–7.
88. Krain LJ, Atwell JE, Nelson KE, et al. Review article: fetal and neonatal health consequences of vertically transmitted hepatitis E virus infection. Am J Trop Med Hyg 2014;90(2):365–70.
89. Khuroo MS, Kamili S, Khuroo MS. Clinical course and duration of viremia in vertically transmitted hepatitis E virus (HEV) infection in babies born to HEV-infected mothers. J Viral Hepat 2009;16(7):519–23.
90. Rein DB, Stevens G, Theaker J, et al. The global burden of hepatitis E virus. Hepatology 2011;55(4):988–97.
91. Sultana R, Humayun S. Fetomaternal outcome in acute hepatitis e. J Coll Physicians Surg Pak 2014;24(2):127–30.
92. Bose PD, Das BC, Hazam RK, et al. Evidence of extrahepatic replication of hepatitis E virus in human placenta. J Gen Virol 2014. http://dx.doi.org/10.1099/vir.0.063602-0.
93. Mehta A, Singla A, Rajaram S. Prognostic factors for fulminant viral hepatitis in pregnancy. Int J Gynaecol Obstet 2012;118:172–5.
94. Borkakoti J, Hazam RK, Mohammad A, et al. Does high viral load of hepatitis E virus influence the severity and prognosis of acute liver failure during pregnancy? J Med Virol 2013;85:620–6.
95. Salam GD, Kumar A, Kar P, et al. Serum tumor necrosis factor-alpha level in hepatitis E virus-related acute viral hepatitis and fulminant hepatic failure in pregnancy women. Hepatol Res 2013;43(8):826–35.
96. Devi SG, Kumar A, Kar P, et al. Association of pregnancy outcome with cytokine gene polymorphisms in HEV infection during pregnancy. J Med Virol 2014. http://dx.doi.org/10.1002/jmv.23925.
97. Renou C, Gobert V, Locher C, et al. Prospective study of hepatitis E virus infection among pregnant women in France. Virol J 2014;11(1):68.

Screening, Prevention, and Treatment of Congenital Cytomegalovirus

Julie Johnson, MD*, Brenna Anderson, MD, MSc

KEYWORDS

- Cytomegalovirus • Congenital infection • CMV diagnosis • CMV prevention
- CMV hyperimmune globulin

KEY POINTS

- Congenital CMV affects 0.64% of births each year and is one of the most common causes of childhood disability.
- Routine screening for primary infection in pregnant women is not recommended by the Centers for Disease Control and Prevention (CDC) or the American College of Obstetricians and Gynecologists.
- There is insufficient evidence to support the use of passive immunization to prevent congenital infection.
- There is no effective vaccine for primary prevention.
- The best means of prevention is through reducing exposure to the virus.
- Pregnant women at risk of exposure should be counseled regarding congenital CMV and hygiene measures.

INTRODUCTION

Congenital cytomegalovirus (CMV) affects approximately 0.64% of newborns each year.[1,2] There are approximately 27,000 cases annually in the United States.[3] Of those children, almost 20% develop permanent disabilities and 1% do not survive. In addition to a significant emotional burden, the annual costs associated with CMV are estimated to be at least $1 to $2 billion.[4] Currently, the only known means of reducing the risk of congenital CMV is by reducing exposure to the virus. However, it has not been shown that educating pregnant women regarding risk-reduction behavior is effective.

The authors have nothing to disclose.
Department of Obstetrics & Gynecology, Women & Infants Hospital, Alpert Medical School of Brown University, 101 Dudley Street, Providence, RI 02905, USA
* Corresponding author.
E-mail address: jujohnson@wihri.org

CLINICAL OUTCOMES

Clinical outcomes of neonates affected by congenital CMV vary greatly. Fowler and colleagues[5] compared outcomes of CMV-infected neonates born to mothers with primary infection (N = 125) with mothers with recurrent infection (N = 64). The only infants with symptoms at birth (18%) were in the primary maternal infection group. Symptoms found in those affected at birth are jaundice, petechiae, hepatosplenomegaly, small for gestational age, preterm birth, microcephaly, and death. Children were followed for up to 6 years after birth, and 25% of primary infections versus 8% of recurrent infections (P = .003) developed sequelae. Sensorineural hearing loss was the most common finding (15% vs 5%; P = .05).[4] Outcomes associated with congenital CMV in the infected newborn are as follows:

- Hearing loss (15%)
- Vision loss (2%)
- Mental disability (13%)
- Microcephaly (5%)
- Seizures (5%)
- Death (2%)

EPIDEMIOLOGY

CMV is a member of the Herpesvirus family. Like other members of this family, after the initial infection, reactivation of a latent infection can occur as can reinfection with a different strain of virus. Seroprevalence rates range from 40% to 83% in women of childbearing age in the United States, whereas seroconversion occurs in approximately 1% to 4% of seronegative pregnant women.[3,6–8] Vertical transmission may occur after either a primary or secondary infection, but the rates are much higher after a primary infection (30%–40% vs 1%).[9,10] However, nonprimary maternal infection may be responsible for up to 75% of all congenital infections.[11] With increasing gestational age, the transmission rates increase, but severity of congenital disease decreases.[12]

The virus is shed in bodily fluids, such as saliva, urine, or semen. Transmission occurs with direct contact. Women at highest risk of infection are those that are exposed to the saliva or urine of young children.[13] Up to 45% of seronegative parents with young children shedding the CMV virus become infected.[14]

BIOLOGY OF CYTOMEGALOVIRUS INFECTION

Once infected with CMV, the incubation period is approximately 1 month. After 1 month, symptoms and/or viremia are present and the virus is shed in multiple bodily fluids. CMV-specific IgM antibodies peak 1 to 3 months after a primary infection and may be detected for up to a year.[15] CMV IgG antibodies are produced during the first few months of infection. They are initially of low avidity and after a maturation process, they have a high avidity. High IgM levels in combination with a low IgG avidity assay is representative of a recent infection (within the past 3 months).[16] The true mechanism of transplacental infection is unknown. One plausible hypothesis is the transport of nonneutralizing IgG-virion particles by transcytosis.[17]

DIAGNOSIS

Routine screening for primary infection in pregnant women is not recommended by the Centers for Disease Control and Prevention (CDC) or the American College of

Obstetricians and Gynecologists. Current CDC recommendations are to screen only those women with a mononucleosis syndrome with a mild hepatitis.[18–20] Although seroconversion is the gold standard for diagnosis, many women do not have initial negative serology because screening is not recommended. Diagnosis of a primary infection begins with drawing titers of CMV-specific IgG and IgM. Positive IgM alone does not diagnose primary infection. Less than 10% to 30% of women with a positive IgM have a primary infection.[21,22] Diagnosis is confirmed with either seroconversion or a positive IgM with a low-avidity IgG. The sensitivity of a positive IgM in combination with a low-avidity IgG is 92% compared with serial serology.[23]

With confirmation of acute maternal infection, fetal infection may be confirmed with culture and polymerase chain reaction (PCR) of amniotic fluid. Liesnard and colleagues[24] prospectively followed 239 fetuses at risk for congenital CMV infection. Fetal condition was evaluated with PCR and cultures obtained by amniocentesis and cordocentesis. The single most sensitive test was PCR of amniotic fluid (78% sensitivity). The addition of fetal blood testing increased the sensitivity to 80%, which must be balanced with the increased risk associated with this procedure. In 8 of the 44 cases, the PCR was positive, but the virus did not grow in culture. Furthermore, the authors note that all antenatal diagnoses were made after 21 weeks gestation with a lapse of at least 7 weeks after positive maternal serology. Azam and colleagues[25] also performed a prospective study evaluating the diagnosis of congenital CMV in at-risk fetuses and came to a similar conclusion. The sensitivity and specificity of amniocentesis was 77% and 100%, respectively, with no significant improvement in accuracy with the addition of cordocentesis. A positive amniotic fluid culture was not able to predict the severity of neonatal disease. **Fig. 1** provides a complete algorithm.

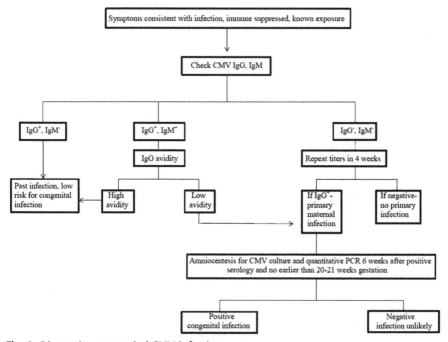

Fig. 1. Diagnosing congenital CMV infection.

Ultrasound may be used as an adjunct and a detailed survey should be performed in addition to amniocentesis. In the setting of a maternal infection and unknown fetal status, ultrasound abnormalities only predict symptomatic infection in 30% of cases.[26] When fetal infection is confirmed, abnormal ultrasound findings are present in 15% to 52% of fetuses.[26,27] A more complete list of ultrasound findings is listed in **Table 1**.

PREVENTION

Currently, there is no effective vaccine to prevent congenital CMV. The Institute of Medicine has ranked the development of a CMV vaccine as a highest priority, and research is ongoing. There are no current vaccines in phase 3 trial. A recent randomized trial of a recombinant CMV envelope glycoprotein B vaccine in seronegative women showed 50% efficacy, but did not give long-term protection.[28,29] One major hurdle for vaccination is the high rate of reinfection with a new strain or reactivation of a latent strain in a large percentage of women.

Without an effective vaccine, the only known means of primary prevention is to reduce exposure to the virus. To reduce exposure, patients and providers need to be educated regarding CMV and the associated risks. In a sample of about 4000 people, Cannon and colleagues[13] found that only 3% of women and 7% of men had even heard of congenital CMV. In addition, fewer than half (44%) of obstetricians surveyed by American College of Obstetricians and Gynecologists counsel their pregnant patients about CMV prevention.[30]

There is preliminary evidence demonstrating that in women who are pregnant, education with assessment of adherence may be effective at reducing seroconversion. Adler and colleagues[31] prospectively studied 166 seronegative women with young children (<3 years of age). The control group received basic CMV information, whereas two intervention groups received CMV information, extensive hygiene education, and serologic status. There was no difference in the rate of seroconversion in the control and intervention groups. However, women that were attempting pregnancy in the intervention group (and had a child shedding CMV virus) had a higher rate of seroconversion than those already pregnant in the same group (10 of 24 vs 1

Table 1	
Sonographic findings associated with congenital CMV	
Sonographic Findings	**%**
Any ultrasound finding	15–52
Intrauterine growth restriction	10
Cerebral ventriculomegaly	3–5
Microcephaly	10
Intracranial calcifications	1–18
Ascites	4
Hydrops fetalis	1
Fluid abnormalities	8
Echogenic bowel	5–26
Liver calcifications	3

Data from Benoist G, Salomon L, Jacquemard F, et al. The prognostic value of ultrasound abnormalities and biologic parameters in blood of fetuses infected with cytomegalovirus. BJOG 2008;115:823–9; and Guerra B, Simonazzi G, Puccetti C, et al. Ultrasound prediction of symptomatic congenital cytomegalovirus infection. Am J Obstet Gynecol 2008;198:380.e1–7.

of 17; P = .008). In addition, there is an ongoing randomized control trial evaluating whether knowledge of serum screening results and behavioral intervention will increase compliance with hygiene measures to reduce exposure to the virus (Clinicaltrials.gov number NCT01819519). Current recommendations from the CDC to prevent exposure in pregnant women are as follows:

- Wash your hands with soap and water after changing diapers, feeding a child, handling toys, wiping a child's nose or drool
- Do not share food, drinks, or eating utensils with young children
- Do not share a toothbrush
- Do not put a pacifier in your mouth
- Avoid contact with saliva
- Clean toys, countertops, or other surfaces that come into contact with a child's urine or saliva

INTERVENTION

Currently, therapies for treatment of congenital CMV are in the experimental stage. A prospective cohort study by Nigro and colleagues[32] demonstrated possible efficacy of CMV hyperimmune globulin (HIG) in treating congenital infection. A recently completed randomized placebo-controlled trial concluded that treatment of primary maternal infection with CMV HIG did not affect the rate of congenital infection. Of the women in the HIG group, 30% were infected and in the placebo group, 44% were infected.[33] It may be that this study of 124 women was underpowered to detect a smaller effect than was originally estimated. In addition, this trial reported a possible higher rate of preterm birth among those who received HIG. Given this, HIG for the prevention of congenital CMV should not be administered outside of a clinical trial. There are currently two ongoing randomized trials evaluating the efficacy of CMV HIG and prevention of congenital infection that will contribute to this body of evidence (ClinicalTrials.gov number NCT01376778).[34]

SUMMARY

Congenital CMV is an important pathogen as a major cause of hearing loss, visual loss, and impairment in newborns. Although an effective vaccine is a high priority, it does not seem that this will come to fruition in the near future. With the two ongoing trials evaluating the effectiveness of CMV HIG, it may be possible to reduce the risk of placental transmission with this treatment.

In 2012, a CMV Vaccine Workshop was held in Bethesda, Maryland and attended by a diverse group of representatives in the health care field.[29] This working group identified several areas in need of future research, besides vaccine development. Some areas identified for further study included

- A standardized definition of congenital CMV disease
- Better characterization of CMV-associated fetal loss
- Further defining predictors of CMV outcomes
- Further study regarding the contribution of primary and nonprimary infection to the overall burden of disease
- Improved assays to detect infection in seropositive women
- Increase public awareness

Currently the best known method of prevention is through reducing exposure in women at risk. With such low rates of knowledge regarding CMV infection in the general population, education is paramount. Obstetric providers may contribute by risk assessment of patients and educating those at high risk of exposure.

REFERENCES

1. Kenneson A, Cannon MJ. Review and metanalysis of the epidemiology of congenital cytomegalovirus (CMV) infection. Rev Med Virol 2007;17:253–76.
2. Dollard SC, Grosse SD, Ross DS. New estimates of the prevalence of neurological and sensory sequelae and mortality associated with congenital cytomegalovirus infection. Rev Med Virol 2007;17:355–63.
3. Colugnati F, Staras S, Dollard SC, et al. Incidence of cytomegalovirus infection among the general population and pregnant women in the United States. BMC Infect Dis 2007;7:71.
4. Cannon MJ, Davis KF. Washing our hands of the congenital cytomegalovirus disease epidemic. BMC Public Health 2005;5:70.
5. Fowler KB, Stagno S, Pass RF, et al. The outcome of congenital cytomegalovirus infection in relation to maternal antibody status. N Engl J Med 1992;326:663–7.
6. Gaytant MA, Steegers EA, Semmekrot BA, et al. Congenital cytomegalovirus infection: review of the epidemiology and outcome. Obstet Gynecol Surv 2002; 57:245–56.
7. Stagno S, Pass RF, Dworsky ME, et al. Maternal cytomegalovirus and perinatal transmission. Clin Obstet Gynecol 1982;25:563–76.
8. Ludwig A, Henge H. Epidemiological impact and disease burden of congenital cytomegalovirus infection in Europe. Euro Surveill 2009;14:1–7.
9. Fowler KB, Stagno S, Pass RF. Maternal immunity and prevention of congenital cytomegalovirus infection. JAMA 2003;289:1008–11.
10. Stagno S, Pass RF, Cloud G, et al. Primary cytomegalovirus infection in pregnancy: incidence, transmission to fetus, and clinical outcome. JAMA 1986;256:1904–8.
11. Wang C, Zhang X, Bialek S, et al. Attribution of congenital cytomegalovirus infection to primary versus non-primary maternal infection. Clin Infect Dis 2011;52:e11.
12. Enders G, Daiminger A, Bader U, et al. Intrauterine transmission and clinical outcome of 248 pregnancies with primary cytomegalovirus infection in relation to gestational age. J Clin Virol 2011;52(3):244–6.
13. Cannon MJ, Westbrook K, Levis D, et al. Awareness of and behaviors related to child-to-mother transmission of cytomegalovirus. Prev Med 2012;54:351–7.
14. Pass RF, Hutto C, Ricks R, et al. Increased rate of cytomegalovirus infection among parents of children attending day-care centers. N Engl J Med 1986; 314:1414–8.
15. Munro SC, Hall B, Whybin LR, et al. Diagnosis of and screening for cytomegalovirus infection in pregnant women. J Clin Microbiol 2005;43(9):4713.
16. Revello MG, Gerna G. Diagnosis and management of human cytomegalovirus infection in the mother, fetus, and newborn infant. Clin Microbiol Rev 2002; 15(4):680–715.
17. Maidji E, McDonagh S, Genbacer O, et al. Maternal antibodies enhance or prevent cytomegalovirus infection in the placenta by neonatal Fc receptor-mediated transcytosis. Am J Pathol 2006;168(4):1210–26.
18. American College of Obstetricians and Gynecologists clinical management guidelines for obstetricians-gynecologists, perinatal viral and parasitic infections. Washington, DC: American College of Obstetricians and Gynecologists. ACOG Practice Bulletin- Number 20, September 2000, reaffirmed in 2013.

19. At risk patients. Available at: http://www.cdc.gov/cmv/clinical/at-risk.html. Accessed May 14, 2014.
20. Clinical diagnosis and treatment. Available at: http://www.cdc.gov/cmv/clinical/diagnosis-treatment.html. Accessed May 30, 2014.
21. Guerra B, Simonazzi G, Banfi A, et al. Impact of diagnostic and confirmatory tests and prenatal counseling on the rate of pregnancy termination among women with positive cytomegalovirus immunoglobulin M antibody titers. Am J Obstet Gynecol 2007;196(3):221.e1–6.
22. Lazzarotto T, Guerra B, Lanari M, et al. New advances in the diagnosis of congenital cytomegalovirus infection. J Clin Virol 2008;41:192–7.
23. Lazzarotto T, Spezzacatena P, Pradelli P, et al. Avidity of immunoglobulin G directed against human cytomegalovirus during primary and secondary infections in immunocompetent and immunocompromised subjects. Clin Diagn Lab Immunol 1997;4:469–73.
24. Liesnard C, Donner C, Brancart F, et al. Prenatal diagnosis of congenital cytomegalovirus infection: prospective study of 237 pregnancies at risk. Obstet Gynecol 2000;95:881–8.
25. Azam A, Vial Y, Fawer C, et al. Prenatal diagnosis of congenital cytomegalovirus infection. Obstet Gynecol 2001;97:443–8.
26. Guerra B, Simonazzi G, Puccetti C, et al. Ultrasound prediction of symptomatic congenital cytomegalovirus infection. Am J Obstet Gynecol 2008;198:380.e1–7.
27. Benoist G, Salomon L, Jacquemard F, et al. The prognostic value of ultrasound abnormalities and biologic parameters in blood of fetuses infected with cytomegalovirus. BJOG 2008;115:823–9.
28. Pass RF, Zhang C, Evans A, et al. Vaccine prevention of maternal cytomegalovirus infection. N Engl J Med 2009;360:1191–9.
29. Krause P, Bialek S, Boppana S, et al. Priorities for CMV vaccine development. Vaccine 2014;32:4–10.
30. Ross DS, Rasmussen SA, Cannon MJ, et al. Obstetrician/gynecologists' knowledge, attitudes, and practices regarding prevention of infection in pregnancy. J Womens Health (Larchmt) 2009;18(8):1187–93.
31. Adler SP, Finney JW, Manganello AM, et al. Prevention of child-to-mother transmission of cytomegalovirus among pregnant women. J Pediatr 2004;145(4):485–91.
32. Nigro G, Adler SP, La Torre R, et al. Passive immunization during pregnancy for congenital cytomegalovirus infection. N Engl J Med 2005;353:1350–62.
33. Revello M, Lazzarotto T, Guerra B, et al. A randomized trial of hyperimmune globulin to prevent congenital cytomegalovirus. N Engl J Med 2014;370:1316–26.
34. Interim analysis of the Cytotec Phase III trial in congenital cytomegalovirus (CMV) infection shows clear indication of efficacy. Available at: http://www.biotest.de/ww/en/pub/investor_relations/news/newsdetails.cfm?newsID=1025191. Accessed June 3, 2014.

Herpes Simplex Virus Infection During Pregnancy

Alyssa Stephenson-Famy, MD[a],*, Carolyn Gardella, MD, MPH[b,c]

KEYWORDS

- Genital herpes • Pregnancy • Antiviral therapy • Prevention • Neonatal herpes
- Serologic screening

KEY POINTS

- Genital herpes is common, with 22% of pregnant women seropositive for herpes simplex virus (HSV)-2.
- An increasing number of genital herpes infections are due to oral-labial transmission of HSV-1.
- Women with a primary infection of HSV-1 or HSV-2 at the time of delivery have a 57% risk of neonatal herpes infection.
- Neonatal herpes is rare, occurring in less than 1 in 3000 live births, but has high mortality and poor neurologic outcome for disseminated disease.
- Antiviral prophylaxis is recommended to suppress recurrent herpes infection in women from 36 weeks until delivery.
- Cesarean section should be performed if an active primary or recurrent herpes outbreak is suspected at delivery, to prevent neonatal transmission.
- There is an unclear role of routine serologic screening for HSV-1 and HSV-2 during pregnancy.

BACKGROUND

The herpesviruses are double-stranded DNA viruses that include several clinically important viruses during pregnancy: herpes simplex virus (HSV), varicella zoster virus, and cytomegalovirus. Herpesviruses encode most of the enzymes required for

Funding Sources: Nil.
Conflict of Interest: Nil.
[a] Division of Maternal Fetal Medicine, Department of Obstetrics and Gynecology, University of Washington, Box 356460, Seattle, WA 98195, USA; [b] Division of Women's Health, Department of Obstetrics and Gynecology, University of Washington, Box 356460, Seattle, WA 98195, USA; [c] Department of Gynecology, VA Puget Sound Medical Center, 1600 South Columbian Way, Seattle, WA 98108, USA
* Corresponding author.
E-mail address: alyssabs@uw.edu

replication and, can establish latency by replicating in slowly or nondividing cells such as neurons. Herpes simplex virus types 1 (HSV-1) and 2 (HSV-2) glycoproteins mediate cellular infection, and glycoprotein G on the viral envelope provides the antigenic specificity that allows for detection of distinct antibodies for HSV-1 and HSV-2. HSV is transmitted via direct mucosal contact, and results in replication in the dermis and epidermis. The primary infection may include painful vesicles or ulcers in the genital tract, fever, lymphadenopathy, dysuria or other nonspecific genitourinary symptoms, or may lack symptoms entirely. Eventually the virus infects the sensory ganglia and persists in a latent form. Reactivation of viral replication may occur periodically for life. Recurrent infections may have a more mild presentation, ulcerative lesions, subtle genitourinary symptoms, asymptomatic lesions, or viral shedding without clinically apparent lesions.

PREVALENCE OF GENITAL HERPES

Genital herpes is one of the most common sexually transmitted diseases. HSV-1 causes gingivostomatitis and keratoconjuctivitis, whereas both HSV-1 and HSV-2 can cause genital herpes. The National Health and Nutrition Examination Survey (NHANES) serologic data from 1988 to 2004 estimated that 22% of pregnant women were seropositive for HSV-2, 63% for HSV-1, and 13% for both HSV-1 and HSV-2[1]; this was the first time that the prevalence of HSV-2 had decreased since the inception of NHANES in 1976. Of the women seronegative for HSV-2 during pregnancy, 10% will have an HSV-2 seropositive partner, putting them at risk for acquisition during pregnancy.[2]

The most recent NHANES data from 2005 to 2010 continue to show a decline in the seroprevalence of HSV-1 (53.9%) and HSV-2 (15.7%) in adults aged 14 to 49 years.[3] HSV-1 continues to be more common in women (33.2%) and minority populations such as Mexicans (58.3%) and non-Hispanic blacks (39.6%).[3] From the 2007-2010 NHANES data, 20.3% of women versus 10.6% in men have HSV-2. Non-Hispanic black women have the highest rates of HSV-2 (49.9%).[4] There is no clear explanation for the racial disparity in HSV-2 infection, which has persisted over time.

The declining seroprevalence of HSV-1 with fewer infections in childhood in developed countries and the increase in oral-labial sexual contact has resulted in an increase in HSV-1 genital infections in young women and adolescents, which accounts for up to 80% of new genital herpes infections in college students.[5] The declining seroprevalence of HSV-1 and HSV-2 increases the risk of primary HSV infection among seronegative pregnant women, the primary risk factor for neonatal herpes transmission.

Poor Correlation Between Symptoms and Infection

Because of the heterogeneous and often asymptomatic nature of primary or recurrent genital herpes infections, up to 90% of persons with serologic evidence of HSV-2 do not report a clinical history of the infection.[6] Neither a basic nor detailed clinical history correlates with HSV-2 infection by serology.[7] Signs and symptoms are not able to accurately predict primary herpes infections.[8] The presence of lesions has a poor correlation with detection of genital tract HSV by culture or polymerase chain reaction (PCR).[9] These issues create a major diagnostic dilemma for obstetric providers caring for pregnant women who are at risk for primary or recurrent genital herpes infections. While genital herpes is an ongoing cause of maternal morbidity during pregnancy, the real dilemma is how to effectively prevent peripartum herpes transmission. This aspect has been made more complicated by the changing epidemiology of maternal herpes infections (HSV-1 vs HSV-2)[10] and challenges with clinical diagnosis.

SCOPE OF THE PROBLEM: DEVASTATING CONSEQUENCES OF NEONATAL HERPES

Most maternal herpes infections during pregnancy do not result in severe maternal illness, in contrast to the potentially devastating consequences of neonatal herpes infection. Prevention of neonatal exposure to HSV in the maternal genital tract has been the main preventive strategy, as early diagnosis can be difficult, and prompt initiation of antiviral therapy for neonatal HSV does not decrease severe sequelae in many cases. Disseminated neonatal HSV occurs in 25% of cases and has 29% mortality, whereas central nervous system (CNS) disease occurs 30% of the time and is associated with 4% mortality.[11] The proportion of cases with skin, eye, or mouth (SEM) disease has increased to 45% in the era of antiviral therapy (**Table 1**).[12]

Neonatal HSV is acquired during 1 of 3 periods surrounding pregnancy[11]:

1. Intrauterine (5%)
2. Peripartum (85%)
3. Postnatal (10%)

Intrauterine HSV is a congenital TORCH infection (Toxoplasmosis, Other [syphilis], Rubella, Cytomegalovirus, HSV) and may present as cutaneous manifestations, ophthalmologic findings, and neurologic involvement such as microcephaly, hydranencephaly, or intracranial calcifications. Peripartum acquisition caused by viral exposure in the maternal genitourinary tract at the time of vaginal delivery can result in disseminated, CNS, or SEM infections. Postnatal HSV acquisition is from care providers (including health care workers) with active lesions on the mouth or, rarely, herpetic Whitlow hand lesions.[13]

The American Academy of Pediatrics recently published new management guidelines to standardize the laboratory evaluation and therapy for infants exposed to herpes at the time of delivery.[14] Owing to the late and variable nature of presentation of neonatal herpes, standardizing the approach in infants suspected to have the infection may improve postnatal outcomes (**Box 1**).

Difficult to Determine: What Is the Incidence of Neonatal Herpes Simplex Virus?

As neonatal HSV is not a reportable illness in most states, surveillance, monitoring the effectiveness of prevention strategies, and establishing evidence-based practice guidelines has been hampered. Many clinicians and investigators have lobbied to

Table 1
Clinical presentation of neonatal HSV disease

Disease	Frequency (%)	Time (d)	Presentation	Mortality (%)	Normal Development (%)[a]
Disseminated	25	10–12	Viral sepsis, respiratory failure, hepatic failure, coagulopathy, ± rash	29	83
CNS	30	16–19	Seizures, lethargy, feeding failure, temperature instability, ± rash	4	31
SEM	45	10–12	80% have a vesicular rash	—	100

Abbreviations: CNS, central nervous system; SEM, skin, eye, or mouth.
[a] At 1 year without antiviral suppression.
Adapted from Pinninti SG, Kimberlin DW. Neonatal herpes simplex virus infections. Pediatr Clin North Am 2013;60:354; with permission.

Box 1
Obstetric provider's role in management of infants born to women with genital lesions at delivery, based on American Academy of Pediatrics 2013 guidelines

For women with genital lesions at delivery, assess maternal viral status:

- Send viral culture and polymerase chain reaction with typing for HSV from genital lesions at delivery
- Order maternal serum HSV-1 and HSV-2 immunoglobulin G serologic studies
- Determine status of maternal infection at delivery (primary vs recurrent)

Data from Kimberlin DW, Baley J. Guidance on management of asymptomatic neonates born to women with active genital herpes lesions. Pediatrics 2013;131:383–6.

---

make neonatal HSV a reportable illness to further our understanding of the modern natural history of this disease and improve clinical care.[15,16]

Efforts at neonatal herpes prevention have been complicated by the high maternal prevalence of HSV-1 and HSV-2 in addition to the low incidence of neonatal disease. The incidence of neonatal herpes is challenging to define, and has been estimated to be 1 in 3200 live births.[17] With 4 million deliveries annually, there are 1500 cases of neonatal herpes infection.[11] Using State of California discharge databases, Morris and colleagues[18] reported an incidence of 12.1 per 100,000. Whitley and colleagues[19] found an incidence of 60 per 100,000 in a managed care population in the Mid-Atlantic and Northeast states. This study used current procedural terminology codes for pregnancy delivery and the International Classification of Diseases, 9th edition (ICD-9) codes, with the caveat that there was no definitive ICD-9 code for neonatal herpes. In Washington state, a prospective study of nearly 40,000 women showed an incidence of neonatal HSV of 30.8 per 100,000,[17] similar to NHANES data, which projected a rate of 33 per 100,000.[1]

MATERNAL HERPES SIMPLEX VIRUS INFECTIONS

Maternal genital herpes infections are heterogeneous and may include primary infection or recurrent infections, asymptomatic lesions or viral shedding without lesions, or serologic evidence of herpes infection without evidence of active disease by clinical or laboratory criteria. Maternal infections are defined as:

1. Primary infection: HSV-1 or HSV-2 is detected from genital lesions without serologic evidence of prior infection
2. Nonprimary infection: HSV-1 is detected from genital lesions in an individual with HSV-2 antibodies, or vice versa
3. Recurrent infection: HSV-1 or HSV-2 is isolated in women with serologic evidence of infection to that type of HSV

Maternal acquisition of HSV-1 or HSV-2 near the time of delivery accounts for 60% to 80% of neonatal HSV infection.[20,21] In a large prospective study,[22] 94 of 7046 pregnant women became seropositive for HSV and only 34 (36%) had symptoms consistent with a herpes infection. In this study, 30% of the infections occurred in the first trimester, 30% in the second, and 40% in the third. Women who were initially seronegative for both HSV-1 and HSV-2 had a 3.7% chance of seroconversion for either virus. Women with HSV-1 had a 1.7% chance of acquiring HSV-2. Women with HSV-2 had a zero chance of acquiring HSV-1. This study did not account for the herpes serostatus of the partner. In a subsequent couples study where 47% of male partners consented to have serologic samples drawn, the rate of seroconversion for susceptible pregnant women was 3.5% for HSV-1 and 20% for HSV-2.[23] Duration of partnership less than 1 year was strongly associated with HSV-2 acquisition (odds ratio 7.8, 95% confidence interval 2.3–25.7).[23]

As most HSV infections in pregnancy are asymptomatic, studies have shown that up to 80% of women who have an HSV-infected infant did not have clinical evidence of HSV at delivery and did not have a history, or a partner with history, of genital HSV.[24–26] Historically most efforts at maternal treatment, prophylaxis, and neonatal HSV prevention have focused on women with a history of symptomatic HSV infections. Among women with HSV-2, 75% will have at least 1 recurrence during pregnancy and 14% will have prodromal symptoms or genital tract lesions at delivery.[27,28] Of interest, women with HSV-1 are at low risk for recurrence in the genital tract,[29,30] but when HSV-1 recurrence does occur the neonate has an increased risk of neonatal infection in comparison with HSV-2.[17,19]

Rare presentations of HSV during pregnancy may include fulminant HSV hepatitis that has been reported but is rare. HSV hepatitis can be confused with severe preeclampsia or HELLP syndrome (Hemolysis, Elevated Liver enzymes, Low Platelet count), as transaminitis, liver dysfunction, and abdominal pain may be present in both illnesses.[31] Severe or disseminated maternal herpes infections may present as maternal viral sepsis, pneumonitis, or encephalitis.

RISK FACTORS FOR VERTICAL TRANSMISSION

In a large prospective study, women with recurrent genital herpes had a low risk of neonatal HSV infection (2%) in comparison with nonprimary infection (25%) or primary infection (57%).[17] Although these rates of neonatal HSV transmission, especially with primary infection, seem staggeringly high, the absolute number of infants with neonatal HSV in this study was small. Of the 58,000 pregnant women included in this prospective cohort, 40,023 had HSV genital cultures obtained within 48 hours of delivery and 31,663 had HSV serologic testing. Of women with both cultures and serologies available, there were 202 who had HSV present in the genital tract at delivery (0.5%) while only 10 neonates had HSV (5% of HSV exposed neonates).

Maternal antibody status has a significant effect on rates of neonatal HSV disease (**Table 2**). The explanation for this is multifactorial:

1. Women who are seronegative for both HSV-1 and HSV-2 are at risk for acquiring either form of genital herpes proximal to delivery.
2. The lack of maternal antibodies to provide passive transplacental immunity also increases the likelihood of neonatal HSV disease.

Table 2
Effect of maternal antibody status on neonatal HSV transmission

Maternal HSV Status	Rate/100,000 Live Births (95% CI)
HSV seronegative	54 (19.8–118)
HSV-1 seropositive only	26 (9.3–56)
HSV-2 seropositive only	35 (4.2–126)
HSV-1 and HSV-2 seropositive	12 (0.3–70)

Abbreviation: CI, confidence interval.
Data from Brown ZA, Wald A, Morrow RA, et al. Effect of serologic status and cesarean delivery on transmission rates of herpes simplex virus from mother to infant. JAMA 2003;289:207.

3. HSV-2 seropositive women are most likely to have recurrent HSV (lesions or shedding) at delivery but are also at lowest likelihood to have HSV transmission in comparison with women with primary or nonprimary infection.

A subsequent study of women in Seattle, Washington, Stanford, California and Stockholm, Sweden showed increased risk for neonatal HSV infection (odds ratio 19.2) for HSV-1 versus HSV-2,[32] which is concerning given the increased importance of both genital HSV-1 and neonatal HSV-1 infections. To date, targeting prevention strategies on women with recurrent HSV-2 by maternal history has inadequately addressed the populations at greatest risk and does not address the complex pathophysiology involved in neonatal HSV infection.

The relative contribution of each risk factor for neonatal HSV transmission is listed in **Table 3**. Invasive procedures such as placement of a fetal scalp electrode have been shown to increase the risk of vertical HSV transmission. According to the American Congress of Obstetricians and Gynecologists (ACOG), a fetal scalp electrode may be placed if there is a strong clinical indication in a patient with history of HSV but no active lesions.[33] Other procedures such as transcervical chorionic villous sampling may be delayed if active cervical HSV is suspected. Amniocentesis, transabdominal chorionic villous sampling, and percutaneous umbilical blood sampling are not associated with HSV transmission.

The data for duration of membrane rupture are limited[34]; however, for women with labor or rupture of membranes, ACOG recommends proceeding with a term delivery by cesarean section without delay if genital HSV lesions or prodromal symptoms are present in a woman with recurrent HSV.[33] In women with preterm premature rupture of membranes (PPROM), there are insufficient data regarding timing of delivery, weighing the risks of HSV and prematurity.[33] One small study of women (N = 29) with recurrent HSV lesions and PPROM expectantly managed from 25 to 31 weeks did not show any cases of neonatal herpes transmission.[35] Management of primary HSV infection and PPROM may have to be individualized based on clinical factors, including gestational age.[36]

Additional risk factors for neonatal herpes include parental age. Women at greatest risk for a having a neonate with HSV are younger than 25 years and have young partners (<20 years old).[37]

Table 3 Risk factors for neonatal HSV transmission	
Risk Factor	**aOR (95% CI)**
Presence of HSV in maternal genital tract	346 (125–956)
Type of infection (primary vs recurrent)	59 (6.7–525)[a]
Type of HSV (HSV-1 vs HSV-2)	35 (3.6–335)[a]
Maternal antibody status	see **Table 2**
Delivery mode (cesarean vs vaginal delivery)	0.14 (0.14–1.26)[a]
Duration of membrane rupture	N/A
Integrity of cutaneous barrier (fetal scalp electrode or instrumentation)	3.5 (0.6–19)[a]

Abbreviations: aOR, adjusted odds ratio; CI, confidence interval; N/A, no data available.
[a] Odds ratios were adjusted for first episode versus reactivation HSV.
Data from Brown ZA, Wald A, Morrow RA, et al. Effect of serologic status and cesarean delivery on transmission rates of herpes simplex virus from mother to infant. JAMA 2003;289:206.

DIAGNOSIS OF GENITAL HERPES

There are several methods available for direct HSV testing. PCR testing of a lesion, cerebrospinal fluid, or tissue/fluid is rapid, highly sensitive, and identifies type-specific lesions, but may have limited availability or excessive cost. Culture is the historical gold standard, and can differentiate HSV type into vesicles, pustules, and ulcers, but has lower sensitivity and is less useful in detecting asymptomatic shedding. Women with symptoms concerning for HSV should have viral identification by PCR/culture and HSV serologic testing to determine whether the infection is primary or recurrent.

Type-specific antibodies will develop within a few weeks of initial infection, and persist indefinitely. Historically, early type-specific serologic tests could not accurately discriminate between HSV-1 and HSV-2 antibodies. Newer glycoprotein G (gG)-based assays allow for type-specific testing and can be requested by the ordering obstetric provider. The sensitivity of the gG assay for HSV-2 antibody is 80% to 98%, with specificity of greater than 96%.[38] Repeat or confirmatory testing may be indicated, especially with recent HSV acquisition. Immunoglobulin M tests are not recommended, as they are not type-specific and may be positive with recurrent HSV-2 lesions.

Although not widely in use, point-of-care and rapid tests have been developed from serum or capillary blood for HSV antibodies and HSV PCR.[39] Avidity testing may provide additional information in women with concern for primary genital herpes. HSV-1 and HSV-2 antibody avidity increases over time after herpes virus acquisition. Low antibody avidity has been associated with the risk of HSV transmission to the neonate,[40] but this testing is not widely available.

TREATMENT OF HERPES SIMPLEX VIRUS EPISODES IN PREGNANCY

There are 3 Food and Drug Administration category B antiviral medications for the treatment of herpes: acyclovir, famciclovir, and valacyclovir. Acyclovir is a nucleoside analogue that inhibits the viral thymidine kinase and DNA replication in infected cells. It has low bioavailability and requires frequent dosing. Valacyclovir is a prodrug that is rapidly metabolized to acyclovir with improved bioavailability, and requires less frequent dosing. There are minimal data on the use of famciclovir in pregnancy, but there is no documented fetal or embryonic teratogenicity from these medications. Neutropenia may be a side effect of neonatal treatment with acyclovir, but this has not been reported with maternal prophylactic therapy.[12]

Treatment regimens for HSV in pregnancy are listed in **Table 4**. The frequent dosing of acyclovir may limit compliance. Both acyclovir and valacyclovir are now generically

Table 4
Antiviral medications for HSV in pregnancy

Indication	Acyclovir	Valacyclovir
Primary or first-episode	400 mg PO TID for 7–10 d	1 g PO BID for 7–10 d
Symptomatic recurrent episode	400 mg PO TID for 5 d 800 mg PO BID for 5 d	500 mg PO BID for 3 d 1 g PO daily for 5 d
Prophylaxis or suppression	400 mg PO TID from 36 wk until delivery	500 mg PO BID from 36 wk until delivery

Abbreviations: BID, twice daily; PO, by mouth; TID, 3 times daily.
Data from ACOG Committee on Practice Bulletins. ACOG Practice Bulletin. Clinical management guidelines for obstetrician-gynecologists. No. 82 June 2007. Management of herpes in pregnancy. Obstet Gynecol 2007;109:1492.

manufactured, but the local cost may still be higher for valacyclovir for women without insurance. These factors could influence practitioners' prescribing habits and patient compliance. For rare disseminated or severe HSV disease requiring hospitalization because of CNS manifestations, pneumonitis, or hepatitis, intravenous acyclovir, 5 to 10 mg/kg every 8 hours for 2 to 7 days followed by prolonged oral therapy, is indicated.

Both acyclovir and valacyclovir are safe during breastfeeding. Genital herpes is not a contraindication to breastfeeding. If a woman has vesicular or ulcerative lesions on the breast, areola, and nipple, a swab should be performed for HSV PCR and type-specific culture. HSV mastitis is a rare contraindication to breastfeeding, and women should avoid breastfeeding on the affected breast while active lesions are present.

PREVENTION: HOW DO WE REDUCE THE RISK OF NEONATAL HERPES SIMPLEX VIRUS?

There are several nonmodifiable risk factors for neonatal HSV, including maternal genital herpes history before pregnancy. To minimize the rare but potentially catastrophic occurrence of neonatal herpes infection, several evidence-based inventions must be considered:

1. Viral suppression
2. Physical examination/cesarean section at time of labor
3. Postnatal assessment and treatment of neonates
4. Serologic screening of pregnant women

Maternal Viral Suppression

The 2008 Cochrane review[41] of antiviral prophylaxis during pregnancy evaluated 7 randomized controlled trials (N = 1249), and included 5 studies of acyclovir[28,42–45] and 2 studies of valacyclovir.[27,46] There were no cases of neonatal herpes in the treatment or placebo groups in these studies. Although the meta-analysis could not comment on a reduction in neonatal HSV disease, it demonstrated a reduction in genital tract HSV at the time of delivery, symptomatic recurrence at delivery, and cesarean section for genital herpes (**Table 5**). In addition, several cost-effectiveness studies have shown that antiviral suppression with acyclovir is cost-effective for women with recurrent genital herpes over a wide range of assumptions.[47–49]

Role of Cesarean Section with Acute or Suspected Herpes Simplex Virus Lesion

Cesarean section is effective at decreasing HSV transmission.[17] For women with active genital lesions or prodromal symptoms on admission in labor, ACOG and the Society of

Table 5
Cochrane meta-analysis of antiviral prophylaxis during pregnancy

Outcome	Effect of Antiviral Prophylaxis
Symptomatic recurrence of genital at delivery	RR 0.28 (95% CI 0.18–43)
HSV detected in the genital tract at delivery (asymptomatic shedding)	RR 0.14 (95% CI 0.05–0.39)
Cesarean delivery for genital herpes	RR 0.30 (95% CI 0.2–0.45)

Abbreviations: CI, confidence interval; RR, risk ratio.
Data from Hollier LM, Wendel GD. Third trimester antiviral prophylaxis for preventing maternal genital herpes simplex virus (HSV) recurrences and neonatal infection. Cochrane Database Syst Rev 2008;1:CD004946.

Obstetricians and Gynaecologists of Canada recommend cesarean section to reduce the risk of neonatal HSV.[33,50] European guidelines further recommend cesarean section for women who have a primary infection within 6 weeks of delivery.[51] Unfortunately, cesarean delivery does not completely decrease vertical transmission, as neonatal herpes can occur with cesarean delivery before membrane rupture. Women with history of recurrent herpes should have a careful examination of the cervix, vagina, and vulva on admission in labor. If active genital disease is not suspected during labor based on examination and history, vaginal delivery is reasonable. Although the presence of nongenital herpes lesions can indicate an increase in genital herpes shedding,[52] cesarean delivery is also not recommend for nongenital lesions because of the low risk of transmission, and an occlusive dressing can be used during labor.[33]

Neonatal Screening and Treatment of Infants Exposed to Herpes Simplex Virus

In 2013, the American Academy of Pediatrics published guidelines for management of the newborn exposed to genital herpes at delivery.[14] These recommendations take into consideration the changing epidemiology of genital herpes infections and many of the risk factors that contribute to neonatal HSV disease, including HSV type and primary versus recurrent infection. The guidelines are only applicable at institutions with PCR availability, and require a multidisciplinary involvement by laboratory medicine, pediatrics, and obstetrics providers to apply laboratory results to the newborn treatment algorithm (see **Box 1**).

Role of Serologic Screening

Over the decades many research groups have advocated for routine prenatal serologic testing to identify all women at risk for HSV infection at delivery.[2,53,54] This approach could benefit both society and individuals by decreasing neonatal HSV, cesarean sections for genital HSV at the time of delivery, and genital herpes acquisition or recurrence. Pregnant women and obstetric providers may be amenable to the practice of routine screening for HSV during pregnancy.[55] The acceptability of partner testing ranges from 47% to 78%.[23,56]

A decision analysis by Tita and colleagues[57] regarding antenatal herpes screening cited the lack of an effective intervention to prevent maternal acquisition of new infection in late pregnancy, and reviewed the cost-effectiveness of various approaches to serologic screening. Routine serologic screening for HSV during pregnancy, with or without antiviral prophylaxis to serodiscordant male partners, has been shown to have total cost estimates ranging from US$150,000 to $4,000,000 depending on the assumptions used.[58–62] Education, counseling, and treatment of seropositive partners can prevent near-term acquisition of HSV infection in susceptible women under study conditions.[63] Pregnant women in serodiscordant relationships for HSV-2 were less likely to engage in unprotected genital sex acts, but there was no change in sexual behavior for HSV-1 serodiscordant couples.[64] These strategies depend on willingness of partners to be tested, which can be limited because of personal and economic consequences. Without this information, recommending abstinence or education regarding sexual practices will likely have minimal impact. At this time neither ACOG nor the Centers for Disease Control and Prevention supports routine screening for HSV in previously undiagnosed pregnant women.[33,38]

RECOMMENDATIONS

At present there are insufficient data to recommend the strategy of routine serologic screening for all pregnant women as a means to decrease neonatal HSV disease.

There is unlikely to be a prospective study large enough to detect a difference in this rare outcome in the general population.

A second strategy would include screening rapid HSV genital PCR for women admitted in labor followed by serologic screening to identify women with a primary infection. This scenario would address 3 of the most important risk factors for neonatal HSV transmission: HSV in the genital tract at delivery, HSV-1 or HSV-2, and primary versus nonprimary or recurrent infections. Unfortunately neither the technology nor infrastructure is currently available for this strategy, and further study is needed. Similar to group B *Streptococcus* and human immunodeficiency virus (HIV) infections during pregnancy, identification of women at greatest risk of vertical HSV transmission has considerable merit as long as there is an appropriate intervention such as cesarean delivery or antiviral prophylaxis. The major concern of this approach is that it would result in an increase in cesarean deliveries without the ability to measure an impact on this rare neonatal infection.

The third strategy is to continue the current practice of focusing efforts on prophylaxis for women with a history of recurrent genital herpes who are at lowest likelihood to transmit the infection. This approach is suboptimal, as it does not address the changing epidemiology of HSV genital infections with greater numbers of HSV-1 infections in addition to the declining seroprevalence of both HSV-1 and HSV-2, placing a greater number of women at risk for primary infections during pregnancy.

Vaccination as a method to prevent genital herpes infections may be the best option to limit the risk of neonatal transmission. Development of effective immunizations for both HSV-1 and HSV-2 could be targeted to adolescents and young adults before sexual activity and pregnancy. There is no effective vaccine for HSV-2, but recent results have shown a modest 58% efficacy against HSV-1 genital disease.[65]

There is a complicated relationship between HSV-2 and HIV-1 coinfection with increased rates of HIV horizontal transmission among HSV-2–infected individuals but, thus far, no improvement with HSV-2 antiviral suppression.[66] In pregnancy, HSV-2 has not been consistently shown to increase perinatal HIV transmission.[67,68] Additional work needs to be done to further characterize the relationship between concomitant HSV and HIV infections and the role of HSV in the perinatal transmission of HIV.

REFERENCES

1. Xu F, Markowitz LE, Gottlieb SL, et al. Seroprevalence of herpes simplex virus types 1 and 2 in pregnant women in the United States. Am J Obstet Gynecol 2007;196:43.e1–6.
2. Kulhanjian JA, Soroush V, Au DS, et al. Identification of women at unsuspected risk of primary infection with herpes simplex virus type 2 during pregnancy. N Engl J Med 1992;326:916–20.
3. Bradley H, Markowitz LE, Gibson T, et al. Seroprevalence of herpes simplex virus types 1 and 2—United States, 1999–2010. J Infect Dis 2014;209:325–33.
4. Fanfair RN, Zaidi A, Taylor LD, et al. Trends in seroprevalence of herpes simplex virus type 2 among non-Hispanic blacks and non-Hispanic whites aged 14 to 49 years—United States, 1988 to 2010. Sex Transm Dis 2013;40:860–4.
5. Roberts CM, Pfister JR, Spear SJ. Increasing proportion of herpes simplex virus type 1 as a cause of genital herpes infection in college students. Sex Transm Dis 2003;30:797–800.
6. Fleming DT, McQuillan GM, Johnson RE, et al. Herpes simplex virus type 2 in the United States, 1976 to 1994. N Engl J Med 1997;337:1105–11.

7. Brown ZA, Benedetti JK, Watts DH, et al. A comparison between detailed and simple histories in the diagnosis of genital herpes complicating pregnancy. Am J Obstet Gynecol 1995;172:1299–303.

8. Hensleigh PA, Andrews WW, Brown Z, et al. Genital herpes during pregnancy: inability to distinguish primary and recurrent infections clinically. Obstet Gynecol 1997;89:891–5.

9. Gardella C, Brown ZA, Wald A, et al. Poor correlation between genital lesions and detection of herpes simplex virus in women in labor. Obstet Gynecol 2005;106:268–74.

10. Whitley RJ. Changing epidemiology of herpes simplex virus infections. Clin Infect Dis 2013;56:352–3 United States.

11. Kimberlin DW. Neonatal herpes simplex infection. Clin Microbiol Rev 2004;17: 1–13.

12. Kimberlin DW, Lin CY, Jacobs RF, et al. Natural history of neonatal herpes simplex virus infections in the acyclovir era. Pediatrics 2001;108:223–9.

13. Pinninti SG, Kimberlin DW. Neonatal herpes simplex virus infections. Pediatr Clin North Am 2013;60:351–65.

14. Kimberlin DW, Baley J. Guidance on management of asymptomatic neonates born to women with active genital herpes lesions. Pediatrics 2013;131:383–6.

15. Handsfield HH, Waldo AB, Brown ZA, et al. Neonatal herpes should be a reportable disease. Sex Transm Dis 2005;32:521–5.

16. Gardella C, Handsfield HH, Whitley R. Neonatal herpes - the forgotten perinatal infection. Sex Transm Dis 2008;35:22–4.

17. Brown ZA, Wald A, Morrow RA, et al. Effect of serologic status and cesarean delivery on transmission rates of herpes simplex virus from mother to infant. JAMA 2003;289:203–9.

18. Morris SR, Bauer HM, Samuel MC, et al. Neonatal herpes morbidity and mortality in California, 1995-2003. Sex Transm Dis 2008;35:14–8.

19. Whitley R, Davis EA, Suppapanya N. Incidence of neonatal herpes simplex virus infections in a managed-care population. Sex Transm Dis 2007;34(9): 704–8.

20. Brown ZA, Vontver LA, Benedetti J, et al. Effects on infants of a first episode of genital herpes during pregnancy. N Engl J Med 1987;317:1246–51.

21. Brown ZA, Benedetti J, Ashley R, et al. Neonatal herpes simplex virus infection in relation to asymptomatic maternal infection at the time of labor. N Engl J Med 1991;324:1247–52.

22. Brown ZA, Selke S, Zeh J, et al. The acquisition of herpes simplex virus during pregnancy. N Engl J Med 1997;337:509–15.

23. Gardella C, Brown Z, Wald A, et al. Risk factors for herpes simplex virus transmission to pregnant women: a couples study. Am J Obstet Gynecol 2005;193: 1891–9.

24. Whitley RJ, Corey L, Arvin A, et al. Changing presentation of herpes simplex virus infection in neonates. J Infect Dis 1988;158:109–16.

25. Whitley RJ, Nahmias AJ, Visintine AM, et al. The natural history of herpes simplex virus infection of mother and newborn. Pediatrics 1980;66:489–94.

26. Yeager AS, Arvin AM. Reasons for the absence of a history of recurrent genital infections in mothers of neonates infected with herpes simplex virus. Pediatrics 1984;73:188–93.

27. Sheffield JS, Hill JB, Hollier LM, et al. Valacyclovir prophylaxis to prevent recurrent herpes at delivery: a randomized clinical trial. Obstet Gynecol 2006;108: 141–7.

28. Watts DH, Brown ZA, Money D, et al. A double-blind, randomized, placebo-controlled trial of acyclovir in late pregnancy for the reduction of herpes simplex virus shedding and cesarean delivery. Am J Obstet Gynecol 2003;188:836–43.

29. Wald A, Zeh J, Selke S, et al. Virologic characteristics of subclinical and symptomatic genital herpes infections. N Engl J Med 1995;333:770–5.

30. Engelberg R, Carrell D, Krantz E, et al. Natural history of genital herpes simplex virus type 1 infection. Sex Transm Dis 2003;30:174–7.

31. Brown ZA, Gardella C, Wald A, et al. Genital herpes complicating pregnancy. Obstet Gynecol 2005;106:845–56.

32. Brown EL, Gardella C, Malm G, et al. Effect of maternal herpes simplex virus (HSV) serostatus and HSV type on risk of neonatal herpes. Acta Obstet Gynecol Scand 2007;86:523–9.

33. ACOG Committee on Practice Bulletins. ACOG Practice Bulletin. Clinical management guidelines for obstetrician-gynecologists. No. 82 June 2007. Management of herpes in pregnancy. Obstet Gynecol 2007;109:1489–98.

34. Nahmias AJ, Josey WE, Naib ZM, et al. Perinatal risk associated with maternal genital herpes simplex virus infection. Am J Obstet Gynecol 1971;110:825–37.

35. Major CA, Towers CV, Lewis DF, et al. Expectant management of preterm premature rupture of membranes complicated by active recurrent genital herpes. Am J Obstet Gynecol 2003;188:1551–4 [discussion: 1554–5].

36. Ehsanipoor RM, Major CA. Herpes simplex and HIV infections and preterm PROM. Clin Obstet Gynecol 2011;54:330–6.

37. Mark KE, Kim HN, Wald A, et al. Targeted prenatal herpes simplex virus testing: can we identify women at risk of transmission to the neonate? Am J Obstet Gynecol 2006;194:408–14.

38. Workowski KA, Berman S. Sexually transmitted diseases treatment guidelines, 2010. MMWR Recomm Rep 2010;59:1–110.

39. Gardella C, Huang ML, Wald A, et al. Rapid polymerase chain reaction assay to detect herpes simplex virus in the genital tract of women in labor. Obstet Gynecol 2010;115:1209–16.

40. Brown EL, Morrow R, Krantz EM, et al. Maternal herpes simplex virus antibody avidity and risk of neonatal herpes. Am J Obstet Gynecol 2006;195:115–20.

41. Hollier LM, Wendel GD. Third trimester antiviral prophylaxis for preventing maternal genital herpes simplex virus (HSV) recurrences and neonatal infection. Cochrane Database Syst Rev 2008;(1):CD004946.

42. Scott LL, Sanchez PJ, Jackson GL, et al. Acyclovir suppression to prevent cesarean delivery after first-episode genital herpes. Obstet Gynecol 1996;87:69–73.

43. Brocklehurst P, Kinghorn G, Carney O, et al. A randomised placebo controlled trial of suppressive acyclovir in late pregnancy in women with recurrent genital herpes infection. Br J Obstet Gynaecol 1998;105:275–80.

44. Braig S, Luton D, Sibony O, et al. Acyclovir prophylaxis in late pregnancy prevents recurrent genital herpes and viral shedding. Eur J Obstet Gynecol Reprod Biol 2001;96:55–8.

45. Scott LL, Hollier LM, McIntire D, et al. Acyclovir suppression to prevent recurrent genital herpes at delivery. Infect Dis Obstet Gynecol 2002;10:71–7.

46. Andrews WW, Kimberlin DF, Whitley R, et al. Valacyclovir therapy to reduce recurrent genital herpes in pregnant women. Am J Obstet Gynecol 2006;194:774–81.

47. Scott LL, Alexander J. Cost-effectiveness of acyclovir suppression to prevent recurrent genital herpes in term pregnancy. Am J Perinatol 1998;15:57–62.
48. Randolph AG, Hartshorn RM, Washington AE. Acyclovir prophylaxis in late pregnancy to prevent neonatal herpes: a cost-effectiveness analysis. Obstet Gynecol 1996;88:603–10.
49. Little SE, Caughey AB. Acyclovir prophylaxis for pregnant women with a known history of herpes simplex virus: a cost-effectiveness analysis. Am J Obstet Gynecol 2005;193:1274–9.
50. Money D, Steben M. SOGC clinical practice guidelines: guidelines for the management of herpes simplex virus in pregnancy. Number 208, 2008. Int J Gynaecol Obstet 2009;104:167–71.
51. Patel R, Alderson S, Geretti A, et al. European guideline for the management of genital herpes, 2010. Int J STD AIDS 2011;22:1–10.
52. Kerkering K, Gardella C, Selke S, et al. Isolation of herpes simplex virus from the genital tract during symptomatic recurrence on the buttocks. Obstet Gynecol 2006;108:947–52.
53. Brown ZA. HSV-2 specific serology should be offered routinely to antenatal patients. Rev Med Virol 2000;10:141–4.
54. Baker DA. Risk factors for herpes simplex virus transmission to pregnant women: a couples study. Am J Obstet Gynecol 2005;193:1887–8.
55. Gardella C, Barnes J, Magaret AS, et al. Prenatal herpes simplex virus serologic screening beliefs and practices among obstetricians. Obstet Gynecol 2007;110: 1364–70.
56. Gardella C, Krantz E, Daruthayan C, et al. The acceptance of HSV-testing partners of HSV-2 seronegative pregnant women. Sex Transm Dis 2009;36:211–5.
57. Tita AT, Grobman WA, Rouse DJ. Antenatal herpes serologic screening: an appraisal of the evidence. Obstet Gynecol 2006;108:1247–53.
58. Barnabas RV, Carabin H, Garnett GP. The potential role of suppressive therapy for sex partners in the prevention of neonatal herpes: a health economic analysis. Sex Transm Infect 2002;78:425–9.
59. Rouse DJ, Stringer JS. An appraisal of screening for maternal type-specific herpes simplex virus antibodies to prevent neonatal herpes. Am J Obstet Gynecol 2000;183:400–6.
60. Baker D, Brown Z, Hollier LM, et al. Cost-effectiveness of herpes simplex virus type 2 serologic testing and antiviral therapy in pregnancy. Am J Obstet Gynecol 2004;191:2074–84.
61. Thung SF, Grobman WA. The cost-effectiveness of routine antenatal screening for maternal herpes simplex virus-1 and -2 antibodies. Am J Obstet Gynecol 2005;192(2):483–8.
62. Qutub M, Klapper P, Vallely P, et al. Genital herpes in pregnancy: is screening cost-effective? Int J STD AIDS 2001;12:14–6.
63. Patel R. Educational interventions and the prevention of herpes simplex virus transmission. Herpes 2004;11(Suppl 3):155a–60a.
64. Delaney S, Gardella C, Daruthayan C, et al. A prospective cohort study of partner testing for herpes simplex virus and sexual behavior during pregnancy. J Infect Dis 2012;206:486–94.
65. Belshe RB, Leone PA, Bernstein DI, et al. Efficacy results of a trial of a herpes simplex vaccine. N Engl J Med 2012;366:34–43.
66. Barnabas RV, Celum C. Infectious co-factors in HIV-1 transmission herpes simplex virus type-2 and HIV-1: new insights and interventions. Curr HIV Res 2012; 10(3):228–37.

67. Chen KT, Segu M, Lumey LH, et al. Genital herpes simplex virus infection and perinatal transmission of human immunodeficiency virus. Obstet Gynecol 2005;106:1341–8.

68. Chen KT, Tuomala RE, Chu C, et al. No association between antepartum serologic and genital tract evidence of herpes simplex virus-2 coinfection and perinatal HIV-1 transmission. Am J Obstet Gynecol 2008;198:399.e1–5.

The Role of *Mycoplasma* and *Ureaplasma* in Adverse Pregnancy Outcomes

Amy P. Murtha, MD[a,b,c],*, James M. Edwards, MD[a]

KEYWORDS

- Genital mycoplasma • Ureaplasma • Mycoplasma • Preterm birth
- Chorioamnionitis • Endometritis • Bronchopulmonary dysplasia

KEY POINTS

- Both *Mycoplasma* and *Ureaplasma spp* cause inflammation leading to spontaneous preterm birth, preterm premature rupture of membranes, postdelivery infectious complications, and neonatal infections.
- Molecular detection methods now allow the distinction between the various species and biovars of both *Mycoplasma* and *Ureaplasma*.
- Genital mycoplasmas are frequently found as part of a polymicrobial infection which weakens the association between these organisms and associated outcomes.
- In vitro and animal model systems must be created to establish causality between the genital mycoplasmas and adverse perinatal outcomes.
- Polymerase chain reaction quantification allows an accurate measurement of organismal burden, which may distinguish between colonization and infection leading to a better assessment of the relationship to adverse perinatal outcomes.

INTRODUCTION

Mycoplasma and *Ureaplasma spp* are associated with multiple pregnancy and neonatal complications ranging from preterm labor to postpartum endometritis, and from low birth weight to bronchopulmonary dysplasia (BPD). In the almost half century since the association between these organisms and adverse perinatal outcomes was postulated,[1] the distinction between these organisms and their effects is incompletely understood. Until the past decade, their fastidious nature slowed investigation. Newer, molecular-based investigation techniques revitalized this field of research, allowing

Disclosures: None.
[a] Department of Obstetrics and Gynecology, Duke University Medical Center, 2608 Erwin Road, Suite 200, Durham, NC 27705, USA; [b] Division of Maternal Fetal Medicine, Duke University Medical Center, 2608 Erwin Road, Suite 200, Durham, NC 27705, USA; [c] Department of Pediatrics, Duke University Medical Center, 2608 Erwin Road, Suite 200, Durham, NC 27705, USA
* Corresponding author. Department of Obstetrics and Gynecology, Duke University Medical Center, 2608 Erwin Road, Suite 200, Durham, NC 27705.
E-mail address: amy.murtha@dm.duke.edu

Obstet Gynecol Clin N Am 41 (2014) 615–627
http://dx.doi.org/10.1016/j.ogc.2014.08.010
0889-8545/14/$ – see front matter © 2014 Elsevier Inc. All rights reserved.

exploration into the pathogenic ability of these organisms, particularly their transition from commensal colonization to parasitic infection.

This paper is written to serve as a review of the effects *Mycoplasma* and *Ureaplasma* infection, with particular attention to disease prevalence, organism microbiology, perinatal outcomes, and disease treatment. Although not taxonomically correct, the term "genital mycoplasmas" is used to refer to *Mycoplasma spp* and *Ureaplasma spp* to facilitate discussion. When distinct evidence exists regarding separate species, a more accurate description will be specified.

PREVALENCE AND EPIDEMIOLOGY

Isolation of genital mycoplasmas initially proved difficult secondary to the extensive culture requirements for organism growth. To expand detection, early studies analyzed serum samples for antibodies directed against these organisms using enzyme-linked immunosorbent assay.[2] Although serologic testing increases the detection rate, it is unable to differentiate between previous and current infection. It was not until the advent of the polymerase chain reaction (PCR) that genital mycoplasmas could be reliably detected and easily screened.[3] Further development of PCR techniques, including nested PCR as well as random amplified polymorphic DNA PCR, allowed for increased sensitivity to lower organism counts as well as increased specificity and differentiation of species and subtypes.[4] In fact, PCR detection methods were shown to be superior to culture-based methods for detection of the presence of organisms.[5]

With the advent of highly sensitive and specific PCR detection techniques, more accurate estimates of the prevalence of genital mycoplasmas can be determined. Various studies have been performed across the world with surprising similarities between the rates of colonization. Initial studies on a low- to middle-income predominately white and Mexican-American population in Tucson, Arizona, revealed a 23.5% rate of *Mycoplasma* and a 72.3% rate of *Ureaplasma spp.*[6] These same authors found rates of 50% for *Mycoplasma* and approximately 80% for *Ureaplasma* in an America Indian population.[7] Similar rates were found in a Canadian population, including both family planning and prenatal patients.[8] Luton and colleagues[9] investigated *Mycoplasma* and *Ureaplasma* rates in equatorial Africa and similarly found rates of approximately 50% and 80%, respectively. Another study in Cote d'Ivoire, West Africa, in 2000 revealed somewhat lower rates of *Ureaplasma* (53%), but similar rates of *Mycoplasma* (51%).[10] Finally, a study of healthy pregnant women in Kuala Lumpur, Malaysia, revealed much lower colonization rates with only 18% of women colonized with *Mycoplasma* and 57% colonized with *Ureaplasma*. These studies indicate that genital mycoplasma colonization rates are similarly high across the world. Such high colonization rates make understanding these organism's contributions to the microbiome and particularly their interplay with adverse pregnancy and neonatal outcomes of the greatest importance (**Box 1**).

MICROBIOLOGY

Genital mycoplasmas are unique microorganisms, characterized by their fastidious nature and subsequently difficult identification.[11] The class Mollicutes is subdivided into 8 genera, leading to more than 200 different species with the majority belonging to the genus *Mycoplasma*. These organisms are derived from the ancestral clostridia bacteria via gene deletion and consequently have the smallest known genome of any free-living organism. The *Ureaplasma* genus is another clinically significant group of organisms.[12] Colloquially these are all referred to as mycoplasmas. They are

---

Box 1
Prevalence and epidemiology—key concepts

- Early detection was based on culture serologic testing (enzyme-linked immunosorbent assay)

- Development of polymerase chain reaction accelerated detection and specificity of testing for genital mycoplasmas

- Worldwide prevalence

  ○ *Mycoplasma spp*, 18%–51%

  ○ *Ureaplasma spp*, 51%–80%

---

composed of a trilaminar outer membrane without a cell wall, which leads to complete resistance to the β-lactam antibiotic class.[13]

Ureaplasma are separate from *Mycoplasmas* by the metabolism of ammonia for energy production. There are 14 serovars of Ureaplasma, which are grouped by 16S rRNA sequencing into 2 biovars,[14] referred to as *U urealyticum* and *U parvum*.[15] Currently, there is debate regarding the relative pathogenicity and clinical relevance of the 2 serovars, which is compounded by the relatively recent distinction between the species. Early literature does not distinguish between the two, which complicates interpretation of the clinical relevance of each of these microorganism species. This may account for discrepancies between studies, particularly involving populations with different baseline colonization rates between the species. Future research must clearly delineate the species in question.

Mycoplasma colonization is essentially limited to mucosal surfaces because the organisms are intimately linked to the epithelium. Adherence molecules are essential to organism localization. These adherence molecules are highly immunogenic and diverse, allowing attachment to multiple cell types, including erythrocytes, neutrophils, spermatozoa, and uretheral and epithelial cells, and are likely responsible for prompting the inflammatory response associated with pathogenicity. Furthermore, they are able to activate complement complex C-1 directly.[16] Finally, secretory products, including ammonia from the *Mycoplasmas* and urea from the *Ureaplasmas*, can cause a local cytotoxic effect further exacerbating the inflammatory response (**Box 2**).[11]

Progression from *Mycoplasma* colonization to infection is associated with an intense inflammatory response. This response is thought to limit the majority of infections to the mucosal surface.[17] This exaggerated response is thought to be mediated by the innate immune system. For example, *M genitalum* is known to activate Toll-like receptors on epithelial cells using lipopeptide expressed on the mycoplasma cell membrane leading to activation of the nuclear factor-κB pathway.[18] Furthermore, trophoblasts from full term placentas are activated by lipopeptide in a similar manner leading to cyclooxygenase 2 and prostaglandin E_2 production. Proinflammatory

---

Box 2
Microbiology—key concepts

- Derived from the clostridia ancestors

- Smallest known genome of any free living organism

- Lack cell wall making them resistant to the β-lactam group of antibiotics

- Secretory products (ammonia from *Mycoplasma* and urea from *Ureaplasma*) cause local cytotoxic effect and inflammatory response

cytokines, such as interleukin (IL)-1β, IL-6, IL-8, and tumor necrosis factor-α are elevated in the presence of genital mycoplasmas and further exacerbate the inflammatory response.[18]

Additionally, Jacobsson and colleagues[19] demonstrated a dose-dependent response between inflammatory markers and *U urealyticum* DNA levels in amniotic fluid obtained from women presenting in preterm labor, suggesting that *Ureaplasma* also prompts an inflammatory response. The association of increased inflammation in the presence of *Ureaplasma spp* is also supported by Kasper and colleagues,[20] who demonstrated elevated IL-8 levels when *U parvum* was documented by PCR in amniotic fluid. This increase in inflammatory mediators leads to the consequences of genital mycoplasma infection seen in clinical practice (**Box 3**).[21]

PREGNANCY OUTCOMES

Genital mycoplasmas have been demonstrated to have a range of effects on pregnancy outcomes. The majority of these effects are thought to be secondary to the inflammatory effects of genital mycoplasma colonization and infection. Inflammation, often caused by bacterial invasion, is thought to contribute to spontaneous preterm birth (preterm labor and preterm premature rupture of membranes [PPROM]).[22] Postdelivery complications, such as endometritis, post-cesarean wound infections and puerperal fever, are associated with genital mycoplasma infection. These clinical entities are discussed in turn.

Chorioamnionitis

Shurin and colleagues[23] described mycoplasma as a cause of chorioamnionitis almost 40 years ago. Interestingly, this group observed that rates of histologic chorioamnionitis are nearly double in the setting of neonatal colonization with *Ureaplasma spp*. They hypothesize that the low virulence of this organism is related to the discrepancy between clinical and histologic chorioamnionitis rates in this population. Chorioamnionitis secondary to *Mycoplasma spp* or *Ureaplasma spp* can be seen in upwards of 70% of women underdoing nonelective cesarean section.[24] Vaginal colonization with *Ureaplasma spp* is associated with histologic chorioamnionitis, specifically because the microbial burden of *Ureaplasma* increases so does the rates of chorioamnionitis.[25] This dose-dependent association supports the hypothesis of ascending infection of *Ureaplasma spp* as a potential cause of chorioamnionitis similar to chorioamnionitis secondary to other infectious agents. Berg and colleagues[26] screened amniotic fluid obtained at genetic amniocentesis for genital mycoplasmas using culture-based methods. Limited by small sample size, they were still able to demonstrate that treatment of positive cultures decreased mid trimester loss, but did not have any effect on preterm delivery. They hypothesized that they were unable to decrease preterm birth because of recolonization. Furthermore, detection of genital mycoplasma with molecular techniques at 15 to 17 weeks by amniocentesis is associated with increased risk of preterm labor and delivery.[27] In summary, mycoplasmas

---

Box 3
Microbiology—further useful information

- *Mycoplasma genitalum* activate toll like receptors and the nuclear factor-κB pathway increasing production inflammatory cytokines, prostaglandin E_2 and cyclooxygenase-2
- *Ureaplasma spp* increase intra-amniotic inflammatory cytokines

play a significant role in chorioamnionitis, but whether they serve as a direct cause or simply as part of the polymicrobial milieu of this process is uncertain.

Preterm Labor

It has long been suspected that premature labor and birth are associated with febrile illnesses. Although the cause of preterm birth is multifactorial, closer investigation reveals that preterm labor is often associated with infectious etiologies. Early evidence demonstrated that genital mycoplasmas play a role in this process.[28] Mazor and colleagues[29] report a case of preterm labor at 32 weeks gestational age in which *U urealyticum* was detected in the amniotic fluid. After treatment with erythromycin, repeat amniocentesis revealed a sterile amniotic cavity and the pregnancy continued uneventfully to term. An observational study of placental culture in successive pregnancies ending with a neonate with a birth weight of 1500 g or less revealed that presence of *U urealyticum* was associated with premature onset of labor as well as a decreased duration of time between rupture of membranes and delivery.[30] Although not demonstrative of causality, a case-control study involving preterm labor subjects with a vaginal culture positive for *U urealyticum* showed that treatment with erythromycin extended the gestation and was associated with subsequent improvements in birth weight, neonatal morbidity, and shorter mean neonatal hospitalization.[31] Taken together, these studies suggest that genital mycoplasma infection may have a role in the pathophysiology of preterm birth.

A recent return to this research avenue supports and expands on these earlier findings. The Alabama Preterm Birth Study observed that *U urealyticum* and *M hominis* cord blood infection was associated with elevated cord blood IL-6 levels and histologic evidence of placental inflammation. Furthermore, the presence of infection was much more common in spontaneous compared with iatrogenic preterm birth as well as neonatal inflammatory response syndrome and potentially BPD.[32] A prospective investigation of endocervical colonization with *Ureaplasma* demonstrated a significant relationship between colonization and preterm labor as well as preterm delivery.[33] By distinguishing between *U parvum* and *U urealyticum*, clinical differences are revealed. Kataoka and colleagues[34] observed that first trimester vaginal colonization with *U parvum*, but not *U urealyticum*, was associated with late abortion and preterm birth. To explain the large difference between high colonization rates and relatively low preterm birth rates, Aaltonen and co-workers[35] performed in vitro studies to assess the inflammatory burden of different amounts of *U urealyticum*. These experiments demonstrated an increased inflammatory response with higher amounts of *U urealyticum* as evidenced by tumor necrosis factor-α and subsequent IL-10 and prostaglandin E_2 production. These studies provide evidence that there is likely a difference between baseline colonization and progression to pathologic infection with resultant adverse perinatal outcomes (**Box 4**).

Preterm Premature Rupture of Membranes

Preterm premature rupture of membranes (PPROM) is characterized by spontaneous rupture of membranes without preterm labor at less than 37 weeks gestation. This phenomenon is associated with infectious etiologies, including the genital mycoplasmas,[36] and supported by the observations of Calleri and colleagues[37] that *U urealyticum* was seen more frequently in patients with PPROM in a prospective observational trial. Oh and colleagues[38] further demonstrated that intra-amniotic infection with genital mycoplasmas caused a larger inflammatory response in PPROM patients compared with other microorganisms. With regard to treatment-based studies in PPROM, the ORACLE trial demonstrated a prolongation of gestation as well as

---

Box 4
Pregnancy outcomes—key concepts

- Placental cultures positive for *Ureaplasma urealyticum* from preterm infants associated with preterm labor and decreased latency
- Preterm labor patients with positive culture for *Urealyticum* treated with erythromycin improved pregnancy outcomes
- Data are suggestive but not conclusive that genital mycoplasma may have a role in preterm birth
- Association with preterm birth may be species specific with *U parvum* colonization associated with inflammation and preterm birth

---

improved neonatal outcomes with erythromycin administration.[39] Macrolide antibiotics, such as erythromycin, have proven efficacy against the genital mycoplasmas and azithromycin has been shown to accumulate in amniotic fluid and eradicate *U parvum* in a rhesus monkey model.[11] Although the differentiation between preterm labor and PPROM in research practice can be difficult, these findings lend weight to the association between genital mycoplasma infection and PPROM.

Postpartum Infections

Postpartum infections can have significant morbidity, including prolonged hospitalization with its associated cost. These infections include puerperal fever, endometritis, and septicemia. Genital mycoplasmas are implicated in all of these infections. As early as 1968, case reports of postpartum septicemia secondary to genital mycoplasma appeared.[40] Further investigation established genital mycoplasma as a cause of endometritis, postpartum septicemia, and postpartum fever.[41–47] There are even case reports of retroperitoneal and post cesarean abscess secondary to genital mycoplasma.[48,49] Watts and colleagues[50] performed endometrial cultures in women with early postpartum endometritis and identified genital mycoplasmas frequently, the majority of which was *Ureaplasma spp*. Interestingly, this was in the setting of polymicrobial infection and clinical improvement was obtained without antimicrobial therapy specifically directed at the mycoplasma organisms. More recent investigation with detection of the various *Ureaplasma* biovars suggests that there is no difference between *U urealyticum* and *U parvum* with respect to postpartum endometritis. However, infection rates are related to the density of cervical colonization.[51] These reports in combination indicate that obstetricians should consider the genital mycoplasmas as a cause of postpartum febrile complications. Whether treatment regimens should include coverage for these organisms is deserving of further study, because there are minimal data and what exist are conflicting (**Box 5**).

TREATMENT

Genital mycoplasmas are unique among bacteria in that they do not have a cell wall, only a trilaminar cell membrane. This lends complete resistance to all β-lactam

---

Box 5
Postpartum infections—key concepts

- Genital mycoplasma are commonly identified in post partum infections
- Targeted therapy against these organisms deserves further study

---

antibiotics.[12] Consequently, therapeutic options are focused on other classes including macrolides and lincosamides. Although fluoroquinolones and tetracyclines are active against the genital mycoplasmas, they should not be used in pregnancy secondary to teratogenic effects.[17] The majority of trials have focused on erythromycin as a treatment agent. Case reports indicate that eradication of *U urealyticum* can be accomplished with erythromycin with or without clindamycin when treatment is prolonged.[29,52] A case-control study of women with preterm labor demonstrated that treatment with erythromycin 500 mg every 8 hours for 10 days prolonged gestation in the patients with *U urealyticm* isolated from vaginal cultures.[31] Furthermore, McCormack and associates[53] investigated the effect of erythromycin or clindamycin treatment on infant birth weight. These investigators demonstrated that treatment with erythromycin, but not clindamycin, prevented low birth weight in patients colonized with *Mycoplasma spp*. This may be owing to the increased activity of erythromycin against *Ureaplasmsa spp* compared with the limited activity of clindamycin.[54] With the distinction between the 2 biovars of *Ureaplasma*, analysis of antibiotic susceptibility between the 2 groups revealed no difference in either erythromycin or tetracycline resistance. In fact, only 25% of isolates demonstrated intermediate susceptibility to erythromycin, whereas more than 15% of isolates were resistant to tetracyclines.[55]

In 1990, the introduction of azithromycin, with its reduced gastrointestinal side effects, shifted treatment toward this choice. Unfortunately, a single 1-g dose of azithromycin proved ineffective in reducing colonization rates of *U urealyticum*.[56] Using a placental perfusion model system, Witt and colleagues[57] demonstrated increased transplacental passage of clarithromycin compared with other macrolide antibiotics. Acosta and colleagues[58] demonstrated eradication of *U parvum* in a Rhesus monkey model using a 10-day course of IV azithromycin that was likely owing to accumulation of intra-amniotic antibiotic. Azithromycin has also been evaluated in the postpartum period. Post cesarean patients were randomized to doxycycline 100 mg IV and azithromycin 1 g orally or placebo 6 to 12 hours postoperatively. The treatment group had significantly less endometritis and surgical site infections, as well as shorter hospital stays.[59] Antibiotic choices to prevent peripartum infectious complications in the postpartum period deserve further investigation (**Box 6**).

NEONATAL INFECTION

Vertical transmission of genital mycoplasmas is well documented. Transmission can occur in utero either via transplacental passage or ascending infection, intrapartum via passage through a colonized maternal lower genital tract, and postpartum via horizontal or nosocomial transmission. Rates of transmission range from 18% to 55% for full-term infants and from 29% to 55% of preterm infants.[60] Vertical transmission rates are not influenced by delivery route but seem to be increased in cases of chorioamnionitis, giving greater weight to ascending infection as a route of transmission.[60] Although preterm infants are more likely to be colonized by *Ureaplasma*, very low birth

---

Box 6
Treatment—key concepts

- Erythromycin (with or without) clindamycin are the best studied and are effective in eradicating *U urealyticum*.

- Azithromycin is less studied, but is likely effective in treating but not necessarily eradicating genital mycoplasmas.

weight infants are at the greatest risk of colonization.[61] With high maternal colonization rates as well as significant transmission rates, neonatal colonization and subsequent infection presents a significant challenge.

Early studies focused on simple mortality effects of genital mycoplasma transmission. Quinn and colleagues[62] performed a case-control study to investigate infection in stillbirth and early neonatal death. They found that almost 80% of cases of perinatal death were associated with genital mycoplasmas, compared with only 30% of control cases. More recent efforts have focused on other aspects of neonatal morbidity. For example, Hamrick and colleagues[63] report a case of U urealyticum abscess at the site of fetal scalp electrode placement and Knausz and colleagues[64] report a case of meningoencephalitis secondary to M hominis. Based on these and other cases, systematic investigation into neonatal morbidity secondary to genital mycoplasmas was undertaken.

Neonatal sepsis and blood stream infections secondary to Ureaplasma is seen in up to 25% of infants with concurrent positive endotracheal cultures and up to 20% of preterm (23–32 weeks) neonates are born with genital mycoplasma bacteremia.[65,66] Conversely, newborns readmitted to the hospital for late-onset sepsis are rarely infected with genital mycoplasmas, indicating that genital mycoplasmas are not likely a significant source of infection beyond the perinatal period.[67] Central nervous system infections have been more difficult to study secondary to the trouble of isolating these organisms as well as the frequent lack of cerebrospinal fluid leukocytosis. Furthermore, the neonatal immunocompromised state and inability of preterm infants to localize infections makes the finding of genital mycoplasmas common in the setting of generalized neonatal infections.[68] Intraventricular hemorrhage (IVH) is a significant morbidity in neonates and can cause life-long effects. Waites and colleagues[68] isolated U urealyticum from the cerebrospinal fluid of 6 neonates with IVH as well as 3 neonates with hydrocephalus. Whether the IVH was caused by Ureaplasma infection or whether the organism was simply sequestered in a large intracranial blood clot is unknown. More recently, Olomu and colleagues[69] found an increased rate of IVH when U urealyticum was isolated from the placental parenchyma. Kasper and colleagues[70] have supported these findings. Further investigation with newer PCR-based detection methods may shed light on this important topic.

Neonatal respiratory distress syndrome and chronic lung disease or BPD is a common morbidity in those born prematurely. Much research and controversy surrounds the role of genital mycoplasmas in the development and progression of these entities. Many studies have found a relationship between U urealyticum and development of chronic lung disease in the newborn.[71] Even in the post-surfactant era, this association persists. The Alabama Preterm Birth Study demonstrated increased risk of BPD in infants born to mothers colonized with U urealyticum.[32] Furthermore, Kasper and colleagues[70] found that Ureaplasma spp infection of amniotic fluid, placenta, or amniotic membranes was associated with increased BPD even after correcting for birth weight and positive pressure ventilation. With the distinction between the Ureaplasma biovars, case reports of U parvum causing congenital pneumonia and sepsis are appearing.[72] There is controversy surrounding these associations. Aaltonen and colleagues[73] argue that, although Ureaplasma spp are certainly associated with the development of BPD, infection with these organisms is likely only a marker for infection. They posit that these organisms do not play an independent role in development of BPD, because when subjects are analyzed with attention to intrauterine inflammation, the role of Ureplasma spp seems to be overemphasized. Finally, the majority of these studies do not comment on rates of surfactant administration, neonatal ventilator techniques, or the use of variable definitions of BPD. Further research in the

---

Box 7
Neonatal infection—key concepts

- Very low birth weight infants are at the greatest risk of colonization.
- Up to 20% of preterm (23–32 weeks) are born with genital mycoplasma bacteremia.
- Neurologic infections/colonization are difficult to study but associations of colonization with *U urealyticum* and intraventricular hemorrhage exist.
- Bronchopulmonary dysplasia is also more common in infants colonized with *Ureaplasma* spp.
  - With distinction of *Ureaplasma* biovars *U parvum* is emerging as a potential pathogen.
- It is uncertain if genital mycoplasmas play an independent role in the development of neonatal morbidities or if their presence is a marker of other infections.

---

setting of modern neonatology as well as genital mycoplasma detection techniques will serve to shed light on the contribution of these organisms to this process (**Box 7**).

SUMMARY

Genital mycoplasmas are frequently found in the vaginal flora across socioeconomic and ethnic groups and have been demonstrated to be involved in adverse perinatal outcomes. Both *Mycoplasma* and *Ureaplasma spp* cause inflammation leading to spontaneous preterm birth and PPROM as well as post-delivery infectious complications and neonatal infections. Furthermore, molecular detection methods now allow the distinction between the various species and biovars of both *Mycoplasma* and *Ureaplasma*. With these advances in knowledge, more questions are created. Future research will need to clearly delineate the species under investigation to allow discrimination of effects.

A large controversy is that the genital mycoplasmas are frequently found as part of a polymicrobial infection, such as bacterial vaginosis or endometritis. This often weakens the association between these organisms and associated outcomes. Future research must use multivariate analysis to distinguish these organisms. Additionally, in vitro and animal model systems must be created to establish causality between the genital mycoplasmas and adverse perinatal outcomes.

Previous research is often unclear regarding the tissue of organism infection, be it the vagina, endometrium, or placenta. Furthermore, newer methods such as PCR quantification will allow an accurate measurement of organismal burden. These localization and quantification capabilities may allow distinction between colonization and infection leading to a better assessment of when adverse perinatal outcomes will occur. This in turn will allow focusing of therapeutic efforts and improvement in outcomes.

REFERENCES

1. Jones DM. Mycoplasma hominis in pregnancy. J Clin Pathol 1967;20(4):633–5.
2. Liepmann MF, Wattre P, Dewilde A, et al. Detection of antibodies to Ureaplasma urealyticum in pregnant women by enzyme-linked immunosorbent assay using membrane antigen and investigation of the significance of the antibodies. J Clin Microbiol 1988;26(10):2157–60.
3. Gallia GL, Petroziello JM, Brogan JM, et al. Development of a diagnostic polymerase chain reaction assay for detection of Mycoplasma hominis. Mol Cell Probes 1995;9(6):415–21.

4. Knox CL, Timms P. Comparison of PCR, nested PCR, and random amplified polymorphic DNA PCR for detection and typing of Ureaplasma urealyticum in specimens from pregnant women. J Clin Microbiol 1998;36(10):3032–9.

5. Luki N, Lebel P, Boucher M, et al. Comparison of polymerase chain reaction assay with culture for detection of genital mycoplasmas in perinatal infections. Eur J Clin Microbiol Infect Dis 1998;17(4):255–63.

6. Harrison HR, Alexander ER, Weinstein L, et al. Cervical chlamydia trachomatis and mycoplasmal infections in pregnancy. Epidemiology and outcomes. JAMA 1983;250(13):1721–7.

7. Harrison HR, Boyce WT, Haffner WH, et al. The prevalence of genital chlamydia trachomatis and mycoplasmal infections during pregnancy in an American Indian population. Sex Transm Dis 1983;10(4):184–6.

8. Embil JA, Pereira LH. Prevalence of chlamydia trachomatis and genital mycoplasmas in asymptomatic women. Can Med Assoc J 1985;133(1):34–5.

9. Luton D, Ville Y, Luton-Sigy A, et al. Prevalence and influence of Mycoplasma hominis and Ureaplasma urealyticum in 218 African pregnant women and their infants. Eur J Obstet Gynecol Reprod Biol 1994;56(2):95–101.

10. Faye-Kette H, La Ruche G, Ali-Napo L, et al. Genital mycoplasmas among pregnant women in Cote d'Ivoire, West Africa: prevalence and risk factors. Int J STD AIDS 2000;11(9):599–602.

11. Waites KB, Schelonka RL, Xiao L, et al. Congenital and opportunistic infections: ureaplasma species and Mycoplasma hominis. Semin Fetal Neonatal Med 2009;14(4):190–9.

12. Taylor-Robinson D, Lamont RF. Mycoplasmas in pregnancy. BJOG 2011;118(2): 164–74.

13. Taylor-Robinson D. The role of mycoplasmas in pregnancy outcome. Best Pract Res Clin Obstet Gynaecol 2007;21(3):425–38.

14. Abele-Horn M, Wolff C, Dressel P, et al. Association of Ureaplasma urealyticum biovars with clinical outcome for neonates, obstetric patients, and gynecological patients with pelvic inflammatory disease. J Clin Microbiol 1997;35(5):1199–202.

15. Waites KB, Katz B, Schelonka RL. Mycoplasmas and ureaplasmas as neonatal pathogens. Clin Microbiol Rev 2005;18(4):757–89.

16. Lin JS, Kass EH. Complement-dependent and complement-independent interactions between Mycoplasma hominis and antibodies in vitro. J Med Microbiol 1975;8(3):397–404.

17. Raynes-Greenow CH, Roberts CL, Bell JC, et al. Antibiotics for ureaplasma in the vagina in pregnancy. Cochrane Database Syst Rev 2011;(7):CD003767. http://dx.doi.org/10.1002/14651858.CD003767.pub3.

18. Oh KJ, Lee SE, Jung H, et al. Detection of ureaplasmas by the polymerase chain reaction in the amniotic fluid of patients with cervical insufficiency. J Perinat Med 2010;38(3):261–8.

19. Jacobsson B, Aaltonen R, Rantakokko-Jalava K, et al. Quantification of Ureaplasma urealyticum DNA in the amniotic fluid from patients in PTL and pPROM and its relation to inflammatory cytokine levels. Acta Obstet Gynecol Scand 2009;88(1):63–70.

20. Kasper DC, Mechtler TP, Reischer GH, et al. The bacterial load of Ureaplasma parvum in amniotic fluid is correlated with an increased intrauterine inflammatory response. Diagn Microbiol Infect Dis 2010;67(2):117–21.

21. Harada K, Tanaka H, Komori S, et al. Vaginal infection with Ureaplasma urealyticum accounts for preterm delivery via induction of inflammatory responses. Microbiol Immunol 2008;52(6):297–304.

22. Goldenberg R, Culhane JF, Iams JD, et al. Epidemiology and causes of preterm birth. Lancet 2008;371(9606):75–84.
23. Shurin PA, Alpert S, Bernard Rosner BA, et al. Chorioamnionitis and colonization of the newborn infant with genital mycoplasmas. N Engl J Med 1975;293(1):5–8.
24. Keski-Nisula L, Kirkinen P, Katila ML, et al. Amniotic fluid U. urealyticum colonization: significance for maternal peripartal infections at term. Am J Perinatol 1997;14(3):151–6.
25. Abele-Horn M, Scholz M, Wolff C, et al. High-density vaginal Ureaplasma urealyticum colonization as a risk factor for chorioamnionitis and preterm delivery. Acta Obstet Gynecol Scand 2000;79(11):973–8.
26. Berg TG, Philpot KL, Welsh MS, et al. Ureaplasma/Mycoplasma-infected amniotic fluid: pregnancy outcome in treated and nontreated patients. J Perinatol 1999;19(4):275–7.
27. Nguyen DP, Gerber S, Hohlfeld P, et al. Mycoplasma hominis in mid-trimester amniotic fluid: relation to pregnancy outcome. J Perinat Med 2004;32(4):323–6.
28. Kass EH. The role of unsuspected infection in the etiology of prematurity. Clin Obstet Gynecol 1973;16(1):134–52.
29. Mazor M, Chaim W, Horowitz S, et al. Successful treatment of preterm labour by eradication of Ureaplasma urealyticum with erythromycin. Arch Gynecol Obstet 1993;253(4):215–8.
30. Kundsin RB, Leviton A, Allred EN, et al. Ureaplasma urealyticum infection of the placenta in pregnancies that ended prematurely. Obstet Gynecol 1996;87(1): 122–7.
31. Antsaklis A, Daskalakis G, Michalas S, et al. Erythromycin treatment for subclinical Ureaplasma urealyticum infection in preterm labor. Fetal Diagn Ther 1997; 12(2):89–92.
32. Goldenberg RL, Andrews WW, Goepfert AR, et al. The Alabama Preterm Birth Study: umbilical cord blood Ureaplasma urealyticum and Mycoplasma hominis cultures in very preterm newborn infants. Am J Obstet Gynecol 2008;198(1): 43.e1–5.
33. Gonzalez Bosquet E, Gené A, Ferrer I, et al. Value of endocervical ureaplasma species colonization as a marker of preterm delivery. Gynecol Obstet Invest 2006;61(3):119–23.
34. Kataoka S, Yamada T, Chou K, et al. Association between preterm birth and vaginal colonization by mycoplasmas in early pregnancy. J Clin Microbiol 2006;44(1):51–5.
35. Aaltonen R, Heikkinen J, Vahlberg T, et al. Local inflammatory response in choriodecidua induced by Ureaplasma urealyticum. BJOG 2007;114(11):1432–5.
36. Kacerovsky M, Pavlovsky M, Tosner J. Preterm premature rupture of the membranes and genital mycoplasmas. Acta Medica (Hradec Kralove) 2009;52(3): 117–20.
37. Calleri L, Taccani C, Porcelli A. Ureaplasma urealyticum vaginosis and premature rupture of membranes. What is its role? Minerva Ginecol 2000;52(3):49–58.
38. Oh KJ, Lee KA, Sohn YK, et al. Intraamniotic infection with genital mycoplasmas exhibits a more intense inflammatory response than intraamniotic infection with other microorganisms in patients with preterm premature rupture of membranes. Am J Obstet Gynecol 2010;203(3):211.e1–8.
39. Kenyon SL, Taylor DJ, Tarnow-Mordi W, ORACLE Collaborative Group. Broad-spectrum antibiotics for preterm, prelabour rupture of fetal membranes: the ORACLE I randomised trial. ORACLE Collaborative Group. Lancet 2001; 357(9261):979–88.

40. Tully JG, Smith LG. Postpartum septicemia with Mycoplasma hominis. JAMA 1968;204(9):827–8.
41. Harwick HJ, Purcell RH, Iuppa JB, et al. Mycoplasma hominis and postpartum febrile complications. Obstet Gynecol 1971;37(5):765–8.
42. Platt R, Lin JS, Warren JW, et al. Infection with Mycoplasma hominis in post-partum fever. Lancet 1980;2(8206):1217–21.
43. Andrews HJ, Dann MJ. Mycoplasma and post partum fever. Lancet 1981; 1(8210):43.
44. Lamey JR, Eschenbach DA, Mitchell SH, et al. Isolation of mycoplasmas and bacteria from the blood of postpartum women. Am J Obstet Gynecol 1982; 143(1):104–12.
45. Boe O, Iversen OE, Mehl A. Septicemia due to Mycoplasma hominis. Scand J Infect Dis 1983;15(1):87–90.
46. Berman SM, Harrison HR, Boyce WT, et al. Low birth weight, prematurity, and postpartum endometritis. Association with prenatal cervical Mycoplasma hominis and Chlamydia trachomatis infections. JAMA 1987;257(9):1189–94.
47. Young MJ, Cox RA. Near fatal puerperal fever due to Mycoplasma hominis. Postgrad Med J 1990;66(772):147–9.
48. Barbera J, Gasser I, Almirante B, et al. Postpartum retroperitoneal abscess due to Mycoplasma hominis. Clin Infect Dis 1995;21(3):698–9.
49. Koshiba H, Koshiba A, Daimon Y, et al. Hematoma and abscess formation caused by Mycoplasma hominis following cesarean section. Int J Womens Health 2011;3:15–8.
50. Watts DH, Eschenbach DA, Kenny GE. Early postpartum endometritis: the role of bacteria, genital mycoplasmas, and Chlamydia trachomatis. Obstet Gynecol 1989;73(1):52–60.
51. Chaim W, Horowitz S, David JB, et al. Ureaplasma urealyticum in the development of postpartum endometritis. Eur J Obstet Gynecol Reprod Biol 2003; 109(2):145–8.
52. Romero R, Hagay Z, Nores J, et al. Eradication of Ureaplasma urealyticum from the amniotic fluid with transplacental antibiotic treatment. Am J Obstet Gynecol 1992;166(2):618–20.
53. McCormack WM, Rosner B, Lee YH, et al. Effect on birth weight of erythromycin treatment of pregnant women. Obstet Gynecol 1987;69(2):202–7.
54. Harrison HR, Riggin RM, Alexander ER, et al. In vitro activity of clindamycin against strains of Chlamydia trachomatis, Mycoplasma hominis, and Ureaplasma urealyticum isolated from pregnant women. Am J Obstet Gynecol 1984;149(5):477–80.
55. Martinez MA, Ovalle A, Santa-Cruz A, et al. Occurrence and antimicrobial susceptibility of Ureaplasma parvum (Ureaplasma urealyticum biovar 1) and Ureaplasma urealyticum (Ureaplasma urealyticum biovar 2) from patients with adverse pregnancy outcomes and normal pregnant women. Scand J Infect Dis 2001;33(8):604–10.
56. Ogasawara KK, Goodwin TM. Efficacy of azithromycin in reducing lower genital Ureaplasma urealyticum colonization in women at risk for preterm delivery. J Matern Fetal Med 1999;8(1):12–6.
57. Witt A, Sommer EM, Cichna M, et al. Placental passage of clarithromycin surpasses other macrolide antibiotics. Am J Obstet Gynecol 2003;188(3):816–9.
58. Acosta EP, Grigsby PL, Larson KB, et al. Transplacental transfer of azithromycin and its use for eradicating intra-amniotic ureaplasma infection in a primate model. J Infect Dis 2014;209(6):898–904.

59. Andrews WW, Hauth JC, Cliver SP, et al. Randomized clinical trial of extended spectrum antibiotic prophylaxis with coverage for Ureaplasma urealyticum to reduce post-cesarean delivery endometritis. Obstet Gynecol 2003;101(6): 1183–9.
60. Sanchez PJ. Perinatal transmission of Ureaplasma urealyticum: current concepts based on review of the literature. Clin Infect Dis 1993;17(Suppl 1): S107–11.
61. Alfa MJ, Embree JE, Degagne P, et al. Transmission of Ureaplasma urealyticum from mothers to full and preterm infants. Pediatr Infect Dis J 1995;14(5):341–5.
62. Quinn PA, Butany J, Chipman M, et al. A prospective study of microbial infection in stillbirths and early neonatal death. Am J Obstet Gynecol 1985;151(2): 238–49.
63. Hamrick HJ, Mangum ME, Katz VL. Ureaplasma urealyticum abscess at site of an internal fetal heart rate monitor. Pediatr Infect Dis J 1993;12(5):410–1.
64. Knausz M, Niederland T, Dósa E, et al. Meningo-encephalitis in a neonate caused by maternal Mycoplasma hominis treated successfully with chloramphenicol. J Med Microbiol 2002;51(2):187–8.
65. Waites KB, Cassell GH. Genital Mycoplasma infections in neonates. J Pediatr 1988;112(1):167–8.
66. Romero R, Garite TJ. Twenty percent of very preterm neonates (23-32 weeks of gestation) are born with bacteremia caused by genital Mycoplasmas. Am J Obstet Gynecol 2008;198(1):1–3.
67. Likitnukul S, Kusmiesz H, Nelson JD, et al. Role of genital mycoplasmas in young infants with suspected sepsis. J Pediatr 1986;109(6):971–4.
68. Waites KB, Crouse DT, Cassell GH. Systemic neonatal infection due to Ureaplasma urealyticum. Clin Infect Dis 1993;17(Suppl 1):S131–5.
69. Olomu IN, Hecht JL, Onderdonk AO, et al. Perinatal correlates of Ureaplasma urealyticum in placenta parenchyma of singleton pregnancies that end before 28 weeks of gestation. Pediatrics 2009;123(5):1329–36.
70. Kasper DC, Mechtler TP, Böhm J, et al. In utero exposure to Ureaplasma spp. is associated with increased rate of bronchopulmonary dysplasia and intraventricular hemorrhage in preterm infants. J Perinat Med 2011;39(3):331–6.
71. Wang EE, Cassell GH, Sánchez PJ, et al. Ureaplasma urealyticum and chronic lung disease of prematurity: critical appraisal of the literature on causation. Clin Infect Dis 1993;17(Suppl 1):S112–6.
72. Morioka I, Fujibayashi H, Enoki E, et al. Congenital pneumonia with sepsis caused by intrauterine infection of Ureaplasma parvum in a term newborn: a first case report. J Perinatol 2010;30(5):359–62.
73. Aaltonen R, Vahlberg T, Lehtonen L, et al. Ureaplasma urealyticum: no independent role in the pathogenesis of bronchopulmonary dysplasia. Acta Obstet Gynecol Scand 2006;85(11):1354–9.

Diagnosis and Management of Group B Streptococcus in Pregnancy

Homa K. Ahmadzia, MD, MPH, R. Phillips Heine, MD*

KEYWORDS

- Group B streptococcus • Screening • Diagnosis • Pregnancy • Neonate
- Intrapartum prophylaxis

KEY POINTS

- Rates of early-onset GBS sepsis in the United States have declined over the past 30 years; rates for late-onset GBS sepsis have remained constant.
- Centers for Disease Control and Prevention guidelines include an option for rapid GBS testing and information about preterm labor/preterm premature rupture of membrane (PPROM) patients.
- Intrapartum antibiotic prophylaxis is recommended for at least 4 hours before delivery, but some evidence suggests shorter time periods may be sufficient.
- Antibiotic resistance, especially to clindamycin and erythromycin, has become more prevalent.
- A GBS vaccine could potentially reduce rates of GBS sepsis in both developing and developed countries.

INTRODUCTION

Disease description

Group B Streptococcus (GBS; group beta streptococcus; *Streptococcus agalactiae*) is a gram-positive coccus with 10 known serotypes. It often colonizes maternal vaginal and rectal flora and can be transmitted to the neonate during delivery. GBS infection may cause significant maternal and neonatal morbidity, including sepsis, pneumonia and meningitis. Neonatal GBS disease often manifests as 'early' or 'late' onset.

Funding Sources: Nil.
Conflict of Interest: Nil.
Division of Maternal Fetal Medicine, Department of Obstetrics and Gynecology, Duke University Medical Center, DUMC 3967, Durham, NC 27710, USA
* Corresponding author.
E-mail address: phillip.heine@dm.duke.edu

Obstet Gynecol Clin N Am 41 (2014) 629–647
http://dx.doi.org/10.1016/j.ogc.2014.08.009
0889-8545/14/$ – see front matter © 2014 Elsevier Inc. All rights reserved.

Prevalence, Incidence, and Mortality Rates

Maternal

GBS colonization of normal vaginal and rectal flora in pregnant women ranges between 10% and 30% in the United States.[1,2] In developing countries, the average rate of maternal GBS colonization is 12.7%.[3] Colonization can be transient, intermittent, or chronic. African Americans tend to be more frequently colonized compared with Caucasians and Hispanics.[1,4] Importantly, colonization does not necessarily dictate maternal or neonatal infection, because it is likely a normal component of the host microbiome.

Maternal infections, such as asymptomatic and symptomatic urinary tract infection, pyelonephritis, and bacteremia or sepsis, have occasionally been reported with GBS as a pathogen. Less commonly, 2% of the 409 pregnant women in a US Centers for Disease Control and Prevention (CDC) surveillance report had GBS pneumonia.[4] GBS infection manifesting as meningitis during pregnancy or in the postpartum period appears in the literature as case reports and is thought to be rare.[5,6] Finally, there is a case report describing development of postpartum endocarditis of the tricuspid valve with GBS after uncomplicated termination of pregnancy at 15 weeks.[7] Maternal mortality from GBS infection is extremely rare.[8]

Neonate

It was only in the 1960s when GBS infection in mothers was associated with transmission to the neonate.[9] More than one half of infants born to untreated GBS-positive women become colonized and approximately 2% of these develop invasive disease.[10] Invasive neonatal disease often results in sepsis, pneumonia, and less commonly meningitis.

Neonatal GBS sepsis is classified as early or late onset. Early-onset GBS disease is typically described in a neonate less than 1 week of life, whereas late-onset describes the disease in an infant from 7 to 89 days of life.[4] The etiology of late-onset GBS disease is multifactorial, whereas early-onset GBS disease is derived from intrapartum transmission. General risk factors associated with early-onset GBS disease are presented in **Table 1**.[11]

Table 1 Risk factors associated with early-onset GBS disease	
Characteristic	**Adjusted RR (95% CI)**
Intrapartum fever (temperature ≥38°C)	5.7 (3.9–8.2)
Previous GBS infant	5.5 (1.7–17.9)
Maternal age <20 y	2.2 (1.6–3.1)
Black race	1.9 (1.5–2.4)
Limited prenatal care	1.8 (1.4–2.4)[a]
GBS bacteriuria	1.7 (0.9–3.0)[a]
Preterm delivery (<37 wk)	1.5 (1.1–2.1)
Prolonged rupture of membranes (≥18 h)	1.4 (1.0–2.1)

Abbreviations: GBS, group B streptococcus; RR, relative risk.
[a] Unadjusted RR; others are all from multivariable model, where main effects included if significant at P<.05.
Data from Schrag SJ, Zell ER, Lynfield R, et al. A population-based comparison of strategies to prevent early-onset group B streptococcal disease in neonates. N Engl J Med 2002;347(4):233–9.

In the 1970s, the incidence of early-onset GBS neonatal sepsis in the United States was as high as 2 per 1000 live births.[12] Owing to our current screening program, this figure has fallen to approximately 0.3 per 1000 live births in 2008 (**Fig. 1**). Estimated projection counts by the CDC for cases of early-onset neonatal invasive disease in the United States are 1425 cases and 63 deaths in 2005. For late-onset disease, there were an estimated 1375 cases and 46 deaths.[4] In general, the case fatality rate for early-onset GBS sepsis has dropped significantly from an estimated 50% in the 1970s to 4% to 6% more recently.[4,13]

Term neonates are predominately affected by early-onset GBS disease, but tend to fair better than affected preterm neonates. Approximately 70% of cases of early-onset GBS sepsis are in term neonates (≥37 weeks).[4] Although only 20% to 30% of GBS occurs in preterm infants, they are 7.7 times more likely to die from early-onset GBS disease compared with term infants (95% CI, 4.9–12.3).[4]

The epidemiology for late-onset GBS has not changed significantly over the last 30 to 40 years at the national level (see **Fig. 1**).[14] This phenomenon is attributable to the multifactorial etiology of late-onset disease and how current national guidelines are focused on maternally driven risk factors and intrapartum management. An antepartum intervention such as a GBS vaccine may benefit this subpopulation of affected neonates.

CLINICAL OUTCOME

GBS infection can lead to significant morbidity affecting both the mother and neonate (**Table 2**). Most studies examining associations between GBS colonization/infection and clinical outcomes were conducted either before or during changes to the CDC and American College of Obstetricians and Gynecologists (ACOG) national guidelines

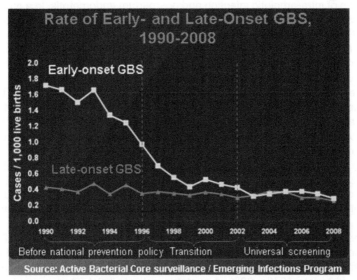

Fig. 1. Trend of early-onset and late-onset GBS. (*From* Centers for Disease Control. Active Bacterial Surveillance/Emerging Infections Program. Early and late-onset GBS 1990-2008. Available at: ww.cdc.gov/groupbstrep/downloads/Clinical_slideset.ppt. Accessed August 19, 2014.)

Table 2
GBS infection and clinical outcomes

Pregnancy	Maternal	Neonate
Preterm delivery	Urinary tract infection, (a)symptomatic	Bacteremia/sepsis
Intra-amniotic infection	Pyelonephritis	Meningitis
Endometritis	Bacteremia/sepsis	Pneumonia
Wound infection	Other: pneumonia, meningitis, pneumonia, endocarditis	

for screening and prophylaxis with intrapartum antibiotics. As a result, there is some variation in the literature about rates of disease and outcomes associated with GBS.

Pregnancy Clinical Outcomes

In a systematic review of studies examining the association of GBS and preterm delivery in women without antibiotic treatment during pregnancy, results were mixed.[15] In 5 cross-sectional studies, where cultures were performed at the time of delivery, there was a relative risk (RR) of 1.75 (95% CI, 1.43–2.14) for preterm delivery. In the 11 cohort studies included where cultures were performed during the pregnancy at different time points, this RR was 1.06 (95% CI, 0.95–1.19). It is difficult to generalize a conclusion about GBS colonization during pregnancy and the risk for preterm delivery owing to the variability in collection times and definitions of preterm delivery. Furthermore, a few studies adjusted for other covariates that are risk factors for preterm delivery. One specific cohort study by Regan and colleagues[16] looked at heavily colonized women during pregnancy between 23 and 26 weeks and found that they were at increased risk for preterm delivery and low birth weight (odds ratio [OR], 1.5; 95% CI, 1.1–1.9) but not preterm delivery independently (OR, 1.1; 95% CI, 0.9–1.4).

Unlike preterm delivery, it is clear that GBS colonization during pregnancy leads to higher rates of intra-amniotic infection and postpartum endometritis. In a multicenter, cross-sectional study of more than 7800 women, women who were heavily colonized with GBS from the lower vagina at the time of admission had higher rates of intra-amniotic infection (OR, 2.0; 95% CI, 1.1–3.7) than women who were lightly colonized.[17] In the same study, the authors showed that postpartum endometritis was higher in women with any GBS colonization (OR, 1.8; 95% CI, 1.3–2.7).

One mechanism of wound infection from GBS is suspected to occur from transference of bacteria through the amniotic fluid. A prospective study identified 6% of bacterial isolates from amniotic fluid at the time of cesarean section as GBS.[18] Others have proposed that the mechanism of wound infection was via increased exogenous bacterial contamination from skin flora, although GBS was rarely isolated.[19]

Maternal Clinical Outcomes

Maternal clinical outcomes refer to conditions that can be both diagnosed during and outside of pregnancy. Pyelonephritis, bacteremia or sepsis, and bacteriuria were the most common clinical morbidities in pregnant women with GBS infection. In a series of 440 cases of acute pyelonephritis in pregnancy during 2000 and 2001 at Parkland Hospital in Dallas, Texas, 10% had GBS identified as the uropathogen.[20] Furthermore, in the setting of pyelonephritis, GBS may be more likely to cause bacteremia.

In the mid to late 1970s, 28% of obstetric patients (49/176) who presented with bacteremia had GBS isolated in their blood stream.[21] The rates of GBS identified in the bacteremic obstetric population over the last 30 to 40 years have substantially decreased. A retrospective cohort study from 2000 to 2008 that showed among peripartum women with bacteremia, only 4% (8/172) had GBS identified as the pathogen.[22] This reduction is likely owing to aggressive screening and treatment as well as general practice changes to perform less blood cultures in the setting of peripartum fever.

GBS bacteriuria is estimated to occur in about 2% of all pregnancies and treatment improves outcomes related to pregnancy.[23] In a double-blinded, randomized trial (n = 69), women with any colony count of GBS bacteriuria who were treated with penicillin had an RR of 0.14 (95% CI, 0.03–0.6) for preterm delivery (<37 weeks) and an RR of 0.2 (95% CI, 0.07–0.53) for premature rupture of membranes.[23] This coincides with data suggesting that any patient with bacteremia who undergoes treatment is at lower risk for preterm delivery and low birth weight neonates. Furthermore, a meta-analysis from 1989 showed that treatment of asymptomatic bacteriuria in pregnancy was associated with a lower risk of preterm delivery (RR 0.65; 95% CI, 0.57–0.74) and that antibiotic treatment reduced rates of low birth weight neonates in randomized, controlled trials (RR 0.56; 95% CI, 0.43–0.73).[24] It is standard clinical practice now to treat asymptomatic bacteriuria in pregnancy owing to clear benefits with minimal risk.[25] Interestingly, it is less clear at what colony-forming units per milliliter (CFU/mL) of growth should treatment be administered. The most recent CDC guideline only specifies that laboratory facilities must report out growth of more than 10^4 CFU/mL[26] and there is some variation in practice among obstetricians.[27] Untreated antepartum GBS bacteriuria (of any colony count) has been associated with chorioamnionitis (adjusted OR, 7.2; 95% CI, 2.4–21.2), suggesting that GBS should be treated in the urine at any colony count.[28]

Neonatal Clinical Outcomes

Although 2% of neonates who are born to an untreated, GBS-positive mother manifest signs of invasive GBS disease, the spectrum and severity of illness can be variable. Early-onset GBS disease can present as isolated bacteremia/sepsis (80%–83%), pneumonia (10%), meningitis (7%), or as a combination of any of these conditions.[4] Both sepsis and meningitis are characterized by nonspecific signs of lethargy, irritability, poor feeding, and respiratory difficulties. A fever may or may not be a presenting sign in the first 24 hours of life. Pneumonia in a neonate typically presents as tachypnea, grunting, and hypoxia. Radiologic features may be more typical of pleural effusions than consolidations as seen in adults. Predictive abilities of laboratory testing (such as a white blood cell count of <5000 or an absolute neutrophil count of <1000) are usually low, especially soon after birth.[29] Unlike early-onset GBS disease, late-onset disease usually presents as a meningitis-like picture.

MANAGEMENT – PREVENTATIVE AND THERAPEUTIC OPTIONS
Diagnosis

Screening guidelines during pregnancy
The ACOG and American Academy of Pediatrics first officially proposed recommendations for screening guidelines in 1992.[30] Two years later, Rouse and colleagues[31] evaluated 19 different protocols for screening and treatment. Their results identified the following 3 strategies as most optimal for the prevention of early-onset GBS sepsis: (1) Universal treatment, (2) treatment based on risk factors, and (3) treatment based on preterm delivery and 36-week culture status. As a result, the 1996 guideline gave the option for either risk-based or universal screening. Another significant change in the 1996 guidelines was specification of the 35 to 37 weeks' time period for screening.[32] Recommendation for when to time cultures was based on a study

by Yancey and colleagues[33] that showed sensitivities for GBS positivity in labor did not diminish significantly until at least 6 weeks after collection. Evidence solely supporting universal screening came from a population study of more than 600,000 women where 54% more cases of early-onset GBS neonatal disease were prevented when compared with the risk-based approach.[11] In summary, current 2010 GBS screening guidelines have been molded over the past 20 to 30 years and gone through many versions (**Table 3**).

Screening methods: swab collection and media details

Sampling of vaginal and rectal regions yields a significantly higher percentage of GBS colonization,[34,35] because vaginal or cervical samples alone are suboptimal and lead to 40% fewer positive results.[1] The 2002 CDC guideline included details on how to collect the vaginal and rectal swabs (ie, the lower vagina and then through the anal sphincter) and later in 2011 ACOG reiterated this in the Committee Opinion on Prevention of Early-Onset GBS in Newborns.[36] Although perianal swabs may be equivalent to rectal swabs,[37,38] collection of this sample may not be adequate in the general population and has not been formally endorsed.

Self-collection of GBS cultures has fairly high correlation with clinician-obtained samples, with 1 study showing 98.4% sensitivity among more than 250 women who self-collected GBS swabs.[39,40] Although not recommended in the current guidelines, this could represent the future of GBS testing.

Laboratory testing with culture media, which at least requires 36 to 48 hours of incubation time, remains the gold standard. Selective enrichment broth (ie, Lim Broth, TransVag Broth, or Carrot Broth) is recommended to promote GBS growth initially for at least 18 to 24 hours.[26] Subculture using selective media is performed for an additional 18 to 24 hours, and colonies undergo extraction for identification and susceptibility testing. In total, to obtain the result by our current gold standard of testing, it is at least 36 to 48 hours of laboratory processing time. Unfortunately, when women with scant or no prenatal care arrive in active labor, standard GBS testing is not practical and most institutions use a risk-based approach to screen and treat these women.

Rapid screening: are we there yet?

Development of rapid testing technology for GBS began in the 1980s. Methods such as latex agglutination, optical immunoassay, enzyme immunoassay, and DNA hybridization included GBS unique antigens or RNA segments. Although these techniques reduced sample processing time significantly, their accuracy was suboptimal.[41,42]

In the effort to improve the speed and accuracy of GBS screening, polymerase chain reaction (PCR), or nucleic acid amplification testing has been intensely studied over the past 15 years.[43,44] The 2 main tests, Xpert GBS Assay and IDI-Strep, utilize primers targeting specific DNA regions unique to GBS and do not require incubation. The most recent versions of the tests consistently have sensitivities of greater than 90% (**Table 4**). Time for processing is variable, but on average takes about 1 hour. Unfortunately, in 1 Canadian study of 190 patients, implementation of a rapid screening protocol in labor revealed a median time for PCR results of 99 minutes, with 81% of patients having results within 4 hours.[45] Even in this ideal research setting, this delay in result would lead to a suboptimal delay in therapy.

Newer techniques are being developing that are hybrids of the culture and PCR methods. They include growth of the specimen in broth followed by PCR amplification. This combination method still takes about 24 hours, but improves sensitivity and specificity beyond most of the current available testing. Data provided by one company marketing such a test quotes a sensitivity of 98.6% (95% CI, 96.5–99.5) and specificity of 93.2% (95% CI, 91.6–94.5). An advantage of this hybrid testing is the ability to perform sensitivity testing from organisms isolated from broth. However, owing to the added broth incubation time, this test is not considered point of care.

Prophylaxis and Treatment

Intrapartum antibiotic prophylaxis in labor

Current antibiotic choices and doses are best summarized by the flow chart proposed by the CDC in 2010, which makes recommendations based on maternal allergies and organism susceptibilities (**Fig. 2**).[26] The most recent CDC guidelines define adequate coverage for GBS prophylaxis during labor. If a GBS-positive woman receives penicillin G, ampicillin, or cefazolin at recommended doses for at least 4 hours before delivery, then the newborn does not need a diagnostic evaluation. Efficacy for penicillin G and ampicillin in reducing colonization have been shown by clinical trials.[46–48] Importantly, these trials looked at colonization and not disease in the newborn. In summary, they reveal a pooled risk reduction of 0.17 (95% CI, 0.04–0.74; number needed to treat to benefit = 25) for early-onset neonatal GBS infection.[49]

Women with penicillin allergy

Special consideration for prophylactic antibiotics must be given for women who have a penicillin allergy. Ideally, it should be clarified with a pregnant woman if she has a type I allergic reaction before labor begins. According to the CDC, type I reactions include anaphylaxis, angioedema, respiratory distress, and urticaria. If the allergy is not type I in nature, cefazolin can be used for prophylaxis. In a population-based study of more than 7500 pregnant women, only 1% of women reported an allergy to penicillin with a "high risk" for anaphylaxis, whereas 8.1% reported an allergy to penicillin with "low risk" for anaphylaxis.[50] Among the women with "low risk" for anaphylaxis, only 13.8% were given cefazolin as the second-line agent for prophylaxis. Clearly, providers are not comfortable giving cefazolin for prophylaxis in the setting of a non–type I allergic reaction.

Interestingly, in the nonobstetric population, up to 20% of patients who report a penicillin allergy are truly allergic to the drug by skin testing.[51] One recent article suggested that these rates may actually be lower.[52] Of the 146 patients for whom they performed penicillin skin testing, only 1 patient had a type I reaction. The remaining 145 patients received β-lactam therapy without a reaction.

Neonates who receive penicillin for less than 4 hours or receive clindamycin, erythromycin, or vancomycin are considered inadequately treated and it is recommended they be observed for 48 hours after delivery. However, if rupture of membranes was longer than 18 hours or there is clinical suspicion of disease, an inadequately treated infant should undergo further evaluation.[53] This includes a blood culture and a complete blood count within the first 6 to 12 hours of life.[26] It is important to use the correct antibiotic and document timing of varying obstetric events.

Unique populations: preterm labor/preterm premature rupture of membranes

As mentioned, preterm infants are at higher risk for mortality from GBS disease. Therefore, empiric antibiotics should be started on women who present in preterm labor (<37 weeks and 0 days' gestation). A GBS swab should be collected at the time of admission and if either labor does not progress or the swab returns negative, the antibiotics may be discontinued. According to the CDC guidelines, a negative result is sufficient for 5 weeks after it is performed. However, recent evidence calls into question the sensitivity of results for that length of time. If a patient returns after hospital

Table 3
GBS screening guidelines over time

	ACOG/AAP 1992[30]	CDC 1996[32]	CDC 2002[8]	CDC 2010[26]
Screening method	Not specified	Risk factor or universal screening	Universal screening	Universal screening
Optimal timing to screen (wk)	Not specified	35–37	35–37	35–37
Population indicated for treatment	GBS colonization *and* any of following: Preterm labor (<37 wk) PPROM (<37 wk) Prolonged rupture of the membranes (>18 h) Sibling affected by symptomatic GBS infection Maternal fever during labor	Any of the following risk factors: Delivery <37 wk gestation Amniotic membrane rupture ≥18 h Intrapartum temperature ≥100.4°F (≥38.0°C) Previous infant with invasive GBS disease GBS bacteriuria during any trimester of the current pregnancy Positive GBS vaginal-rectal screening culture in late gestation during current pregnancy	Previous infant with invasive GBS disease GBS bacteriuria during current pregnancy Positive GBS screening culture during current pregnancy Unknown GBS status at the onset of labor (culture not done, incomplete, or results unknown) and any of the following: Delivery <37 wk gestation Amniotic membrane rupture ≥18 h Intrapartum temperature ≥100.4°F (≥38.0°C)	Previous infant with invasive GBS disease GBS bacteriuria during **any trimester** of the current pregnancy Positive GBS vaginal-rectal screening culture **in late gestation** during current pregnancy Unknown GBS status at the onset of labor (culture not done, incomplete, or results unknown) and any of the following: Delivery <37 wk gestation Amniotic membrane rupture ≥18 h Intrapartum temperature ≥100.4°F (≥38.0°C) **Intrapartum NAAT positive for GBS**

Population not indicated for treatment	GBS colonization by screening culture only	Not specified	Previous pregnancy with a positive GBS screening culture Negative vaginal and rectal GBS screening culture in late gestation during the current pregnancy, **regardless of intrapartum risk factors** Cesarean delivery performed before onset of labor on a woman with intact amniotic membranes, regardless of GBS colonization status	Colonization with GBS during a previous pregnancy GBS bacteriuria during previous pregnancy Negative vaginal and rectal GBS screening culture in late gestation during the current pregnancy, regardless of intrapartum risk factors Cesarean delivery performed before onset of labor on a woman with intact amniotic membranes, regardless of GBS colonization status or gestational age
Screening/testing method notes	Vaginal, rectal, urine or cervical swabs/not specified	**Vaginal or anorectal swab/** specified	Lower vagina and rectum **(through anal sphincter)/** specified	Vaginal and rectal swab/ specified
Special groups	Not specified	Not specified	PCN allergy, planned cesarean, newborn management after IAP	Threatened preterm delivery, PPROM

Highlighted in **bold** are new changes/revisions to prior guidelines.

Abbreviations: GBS, group B streptococcus; IAP, intrapartum antibiotic prophylaxis; NAAT, nucleic acid amplification test; PCN, penicillin; PPROM, preterm labor/preterm premature rupture of membrane.

Data from Refs. [8,26,30,32]

Table 4
PCR or nucleic acid amplification test validation studies for group B streptococcus screening using vaginal/rectal samples and intrapartum culture as the gold standard

PCR Studies	Sample Size, n	Sensitivity, % (95% CI)	Specificity, % (95% CI)	Time to Run Test (min)
Bergeron et al,[72] 2000	112	97.0 (82.5–99.8)	100 (86.9–100)	30–100
Davies et al,[57] 2004	803	94.0 (90.1–97.8)	95.9 (94.3–97.4)	40
Gavino Wang,[58] 2007	55	95.8 (76.9–99.8)	64.5 (45.4–80.2)	<75
Edwards et al,[73] 2008	784	91.1 (86.1–94.7)	96.0 (94.0–97.4)	75
Money et al,[45] 2008	190	90.7 (79.7–96.9)	97.6 (93.1–99.5)	99
El Helali et al,[74] 2009	968	98.5 (94.8–99.6)	99.6 (98.8–99.9)	<75
Young et al,[59] 2011	559	90.8 (84.6–95.2)	97.6 (95.6–98.8)	41

Abbreviation: PCR, polymerase chain reaction.
Data from Ahmadzia HK, HR, Brown HL. Group B Streptococcus screening update: an overview of guidelines and methods. Contemp Ob Gyn 2013;58(7):40–6.

discharge in preterm labor, it is reasonable for clinicians to empirically start antibiotics given the higher risk for mortality from GBS disease in the preterm population.

In the situation of preterm premature rupture of membranes (less than 34 weeks and 0 days' gestation), latency antibiotics typically include ampicillin and therefore no additional antibiotics are recommended. However, if there is an allergy concern or a woman is beyond 34 weeks and 0 days' gestation, one of the alternative CDC regimens should be started. After antibiotics are continued for the standard 7 days, if a preterm premature rupture of membranes patient enters labor within 5 weeks of a negative GBS swab the CDC does not recommend restarting antibiotics. Some clinicians may choose to restart antibiotics if there is high suspicion for infection or solely based on a patient's preterm status.

GBS Vaccine: Where Are We Now?

The idea for a GBS vaccine started in 1976 and subsequent studies showed correlation between GBS titers and risk of disease.[54,55] There are ongoing phase 1 and 2 clinical studies investigating maternal response and transplacental transfer of specific GBS antibodies. There is significant potential for this vaccine to reduce both early-onset and late-onset GBS sepsis rates in countries without screening programs as well as late-onset disease in countries with screening programs. A cost-effectiveness study focusing on South Africa concluded that a GBS vaccine, with an efficacy of 50% to 90% and a 75% vaccination uptake, would be highly cost effective.[56]

COMPLICATIONS AND CONCERNS
Screening Failures

The majority of cases of neonatal GBS are owing to false negative screening results at 35 to 37 weeks. In 2 large population-based studies, 61% to 81% of term infants with GBS disease had mothers who screened negative (**Table 5**). These screening failures are likely owing to the interval conversion of the mother to GBS positive status after her initial culture or suboptimal collection of cultures.

With regard to interval conversion to a GBS-positive status, several studies have challenged the Yancey and colleagues[33] study that showed an 87% sensitivity for antepartum cultures at 35 to 37 weeks. More recent studies found variable sensitivity

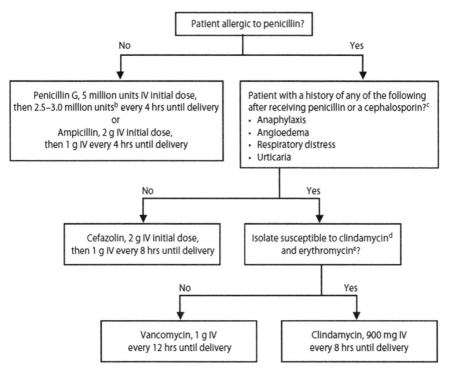

Fig. 2. Algorithm by 2010 US Centers for Disease Control and Prevention (CDC) guidelines for intrapartum antibiotic prophylaxis in women with penicillin allergy. *Abbreviation:* IV, intravenously. [a] Broader spectrum agents, including an agent active against group B streptococcus (GBS), might be necessary for the treatment of chorioamnionitis. [b] Doses ranging from 2.5 to 3.0 million units are acceptable for the doses administered every 4 hours after the initial dose. The choice of dose within that range should be guided by which formulations of penicillin G are readily available to reduce the need for pharmacies to specially prepare doses. [c] Penicillin-allergic patients with a history of anaphylaxis, angioedema, respiratory distress, or urticaria after administration of penicillin or a cephalosporin are considered to be at high risk for anaphylaxis and should not receive penicillin, ampicillin, or cefazolin for GBS intrapartum prophylaxis. For penicillin-allergic patients who do not have a history of those reactions, cefazolin is the preferred agent because pharmacologic data suggest it achieves effective intra-amniotic concentrations. Vancomycin and clindamycin should be reserved for penicillin-allergic women at high risk for anaphylaxis. [d] If laboratory facilities are adequate, clindamycin and erythromycin susceptibility testing should be performed on prenatal GBS isolates from penicillin-allergic women at high risk for anaphylaxis. If no susceptibility testing is performed, or the results are not available at the time of labor, vancomycin is the preferred agent for GBS intrapartum prophylaxis for penicillin-allergic women at high risk for anaphylaxis. [e] Resistance to erythromycin is often but not always associated with clindamycin resistance. If an isolate is resistant to erythromycin, it might have inducible resistance to clindamycin, even if it seems to be susceptible to clindamycin. If a GBS isolate is susceptible to clindamycin, resistant to erythromycin, and testing for inducible clindamycin resistance has been performed and is negative (no inducible resistance), then clindamycin can be used for GBS intrapartum prophylaxis instead of vancomycin. (*From* Verani JR, McGee L, Schrag SJ. Prevention of perinatal group B streptococcal disease—revised guidelines from CDC, 2010. MMWR Recomm Rep 2010;59(RR-10):1–36.)

Table 5 Screening failures			
Study	Live Births in Surveillance Area	Infants with Early-Onset GBS Neonatal Disease (Preterm + Term)	Term Infants with GBS Disease Whose Mother was Screen Negative (%)
Van Dyke et al,[50] 2009	819,528	254	61 (116/189)
Stoll et al,[60] 2011	396,586	160	81 (60/74)

Abbreviation: GBS, group B streptococcus.

Data from Van Dyke MK, Phares CR, Lynfield R, et al. Evaluation of universal antenatal screening for group B streptococcus. N Engl J Med 2009;360(25):2626–36; and Stoll BJ, Hansen NI, Sanchez PJ, et al. Early onset neonatal sepsis: the burden of group B streptococcal and E. coli disease continues. Pediatrics 2011;127(5):817–26.

rates of 35- to 37-week cultures that range from 54% to 84% when utilizing intrapartum culture as the gold standard.[45,57–59]

Implementation errors also contribute to screening failures. In the Stoll and colleagues[60] study, only 63% of term mothers underwent GBS screening at the recommended time period. Furthermore, a recent article by the CDC identified prenatal screening errors as the leading group of errors in cases of affected term neonates with early-onset GBS disease (80/222; 36%).[61] Specific screening errors were defined as no prenatal screen, prenatal screen less than 35 weeks only, prenatal screen performed despite other indications for GBS prophylaxis, and provider most commonly collects non–vaginal-rectal swabs for screen. Laboratory technique was the second most common group of errors among affected term neonates (37/222; 17%), with examples such as failure to enrich specimen and enrichment for less than 18 hours. These implementation failures stress the importance of developing more sensitive screening methods and reinforce the need for education among patients and providers.

Evidence Behind the Guidelines

Some researchers argue that intrapartum antibiotic prophylaxis for neonatal GBS prevention is not evidence based in that the recommendations are not based on adequately performed randomized trials with neonatal disease as the ultimate endpoint.[46–49] Although the current recommendations utilize intrapartum transmission as a surrogate for disease, these data in combination with the significant decline in the United States and other countries that implemented screening programs over the past 25 years precludes neither the ability nor the need for further randomized trials.

Antibiotic Resistance

In the United States as well as European countries there is increasing resistance to clindamycin and erythromycin among GBS isolates (**Fig. 3**).[63] Rates of resistance have been reported to be as high as 32% resistance to erythromycin and 20% resistance to clindamycin.[4,62] Not surprisingly, GBS co-resistance to these 2 drugs is becoming more common. If erythromycin resistance is detected on susceptibility testing, the CDC recommends that clindamycin may be used instead of vancomycin only if clindamycin-induced resistance testing is also negative.[26] If susceptibility testing is not able to be performed, then vancomycin is the drug of choice.

Resistance to Enterobacteriaceae and *Escherichia coli* have been described using vaginal cultures from women before and after treatment with ampicillin or penicillin intrapartum for GBS prophylaxis.[63] Interestingly, significant differences in resistance were seen after as few as 2 doses of intrapartum antibiotics. However, this study

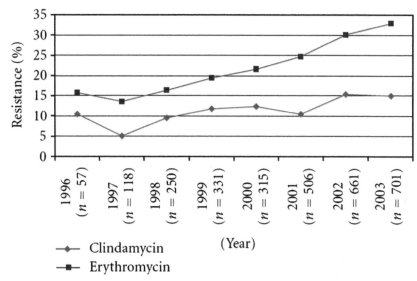

Fig. 3. Group B streptococcus (GBS) resistance in cases of invasive disease (1996–2003) among 2937 isolates in the United States. (*From* Castor ML, Whitney CG, Como-Sabetti K, et al. Antibiotic resistance patterns in invasive group B Streptococcal Isolates. Infect Dis Obstet Gynecol 2008;2008:72750.)

did not include follow-up neonatal cultures to see if that resistance persisted. Conflicting data from larger, retrospective studies suggest either an increase in or no change to ampicillin resistance over several decades.[64,65]

"Adequate" Treatment Time: Is 4 Hours Required?

The recommendation for at least 4 hours of treatment is based on a 1998 study that showed significantly lower rates of neonatal GBS colonization if mothers received at least 4 hours of treatment (**Table 6**).[66] Other studies before and after 1998 have shown that less than 4 hours of treatment may be sufficient to reduce transmission of neonatal colonization. It is important to note that vertical transmission in these studies was defined as GBS colonization and not early-onset GBS disease.

One recent study examined rates of neonatal clinical sepsis depending on duration of intrapartum prophylaxis; they found an adjusted OR of 3.5 (95% CI, 1.3–9.6) for having neonatal clinical sepsis among women who received less than 2 hours of prophylaxis compared with women who received 4 or more hours of prophylaxis.[67] However, wide confidence intervals suggest additional studies are needed to replicate this

Table 6
Percent colonized newborns among women who received intrapartum antibiotics for group B streptococcus–positive status

Study	n	<1 h	1–2 h	2–4 h	>4 h
Boyer et al,[75] 1983	120	31 (4/13)	4.3 (1/23)	3.6 (1/28)	5.4 (3/56)
De Cueto et al,[66] 1998	201	46 (11/24)	28 (6/21)	2.9 (2/70)	1.2 (1/86)
Lijoi et al,[76] 2007	209		12.3 (9/37)		3.7 (5/136)
Berardi et al,[77] 2011	137	5.6 (2/36)	0 (0/46)	5.5 (3/55)	N/A

finding. Other studies have shown effectiveness of penicillin prophylaxis is higher if given for at least 4 hours compared with 2 hours before delivery (91% vs 47%).[68] However, both preterm and term infants who had early-onset GBS sepsis were included together in the analysis. This may have biased the results, because it is known that preterm infants are at greater risk for GBS sepsis compared with term infants and the timing of antibiotic prophylaxis is likely not comparable between these 2 groups.

Additional data suggesting that fewer than 4 hours of treatment may be sufficient for clinically meaningful outcomes include pharmacokinetic evidence. Within the first hour of penicillin administration minimum inhibitory concentration levels of 0.1 μg/mL are reached in cord blood (**Fig. 4**).[69] Treatment with cefazolin and vancomycin have also been shown in pharmacokinetic studies to achieve minimum inhibitory concentration levels of 0.1 μg/mL in cord blood by 30 minutes after infusion of the drug.[70,71] The intrapartum pharmacokinetics of clindamycin and erythromycin have not been well studied.

Ideally, all GBS-positive women should receive 4 hours of intrapartum antibiotics before delivery. However, when a multiparous, GBS-positive woman presents in active labor, she may deliver rather quickly. Based on vertical transmission studies and pharmacokinetic data in these situations, at least 1 or 2 hours of antibiotic prophylaxis should be sufficient.

DISCUSSION

Over the past few decades in the United States, there has been significant evolution of national guidelines for GBS maternal screening and intrapartum antibiotic prophylaxis. As a result of these guidelines, rates of early-onset GBS sepsis have dramatically declined. Current CDC recommendations promote universal screening and intrapartum prophylaxis for GBS-positive women, preferably with penicillin, ampicillin, or cefazolin. The latest version of the CDC recommendations has expanded to cover special populations of women in labor and also suggests a role for rapid GBS testing.

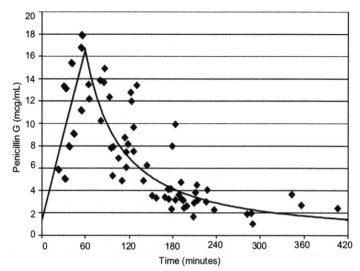

Fig. 4. Pharmacokinetics of penicillin G in umbilical cord serum at delivery. (*From* Barber EL, Zhao G, Buhimschi IA, et al. Duration of intrapartum prophylaxis and concentration of penicillin G in fetal serum at delivery. Obstet Gynecol 2008;112(2 Pt 1):265–70; with permission.)

Despite the success made in reducing incidence of early-onset GBS sepsis, many other hurdles exist to further reduce the burden of disease. Concerns about screening failures with false-negative screens and interval conversions of negative mothers from the 35- to 37-week time period highlight a need to reconsider the methodology and timing of screening. For example, testing closer to the time of delivery may identify more women who are falsely negative with a culture further removed from labor.

Furthermore, improved PCR or hybrid/enhanced PCR methods for detecting GBS will push the boundaries of the current gold standard antepartum culture. Only when the technology truly becomes point-of-care testing, ideally with GBS suscepti-bility information, will it become widely adopted by clinicians for routine screening. However, women with no prenatal care and present with preterm labor or rupture of membranes may benefit from current rapid intrapartum GBS screening.

In addition to better screening methods, better selection of antibiotics for prophy-laxis will reduce concerns related to antibiotic resistance. Reduced exposure tovanco-mycin, clindamycin, or erythromycin could be achieved by better identifying women who truly have a type I reaction to penicillin. Antenatal allergy skin testing may be a solution to help reduce concerns about antibiotic resistance.

Finally, rates of late-onset GBS sepsis have stayed constant over decades owing to the multifactorial etiology of transmission after delivery. A GBS vaccine could reduce ultimately the burden of early-onset and late-onset GBS disease. Furthermore, it may also provide a solution to the other challenges we currently face with our current screening and prophylaxis approach during pregnancy. Many women arrive in labor without screening owing to limited prenatal care and multiparous women may deliver before receiving 4 hours of intrapartum prophylaxis. Prevention is the best cure for any disease.

REFERENCES

1. Regan JA, Klebanoff MA, Nugent RP. The epidemiology of group B strepto-coccal colonization in pregnancy. Vaginal Infections and Prematurity Study Group. Obstet Gynecol 1991;77(4):604–10.
2. Yancey MK, Duff P, Kubilis P, et al. Risk factors for neonatal sepsis. Obstet Gynecol 1996;87(2):188–94.
3. Stoll BJ, Schuchat A. Maternal carriage of group B streptococci in developing countries. Pediatr Infect Dis J 1998;17(6):499–503.
4. Phares CR, Lynfield R, Farley MM, et al. Epidemiology of invasive group B strep-tococcal disease in the United States, 1999-2005. JAMA 2008;299(17):2056–65.
5. Braun TI, Pinover W, Sih P. Group B streptococcal meningitis in a pregnant woman before the onset of labor. Clin Infect Dis 1995;21(4):1042–3.
6. Guerin JM, Leibinger F, Mofredj A, et al. Streptococcus B meningitis in post-par-tum. J Infect 1997;34(2):151–3.
7. Palys EE, Li J, Gaut PL, et al. Tricuspid valve endocarditis with Group B Strep-tococcus after an elective abortion: the need for new data. Infect Dis Obstet Gynecol 2006;2006:43253.
8. Schrag S, Gorwitz R, Fultz-Butts K, et al. Prevention of perinatal group B strep-tococcal disease. Revised guidelines from CDC. MMWR Recomm Rep 2002; 51(RR-11):1–22.
9. Hood M, Janney A, Dameron G. Beta hemolytic streptococcus group B associ-ated with problems of the perinatal period. Am J Obstet Gynecol 1961;82:809–18.
10. Baker CJ, Barrett FF. Transmission of group B streptococci among parturient women and their neonates. J Pediatr 1973;83(6):919–25.

11. Schrag SJ, Zell ER, Lynfield R, et al. A population-based comparison of strategies to prevent early-onset group B streptococcal disease in neonates. N Engl J Med 2002;347(4):233–9.
12. Franciosi RA, Knostman JD, Zimmerman RA. Group B streptococcal neonatal and infant infections. J Pediatr 1973;82(4):707–18.
13. Baker CJ, Clark DJ, Barrett FF. Selective broth medium for isolation of group B streptococci. Appl Microbiol 1973;26(6):884–5.
14. Schrag SJ, Zywicki S, Farley MM, et al. Group B streptococcal disease in the era of intrapartum antibiotic prophylaxis. N Engl J Med 2000;342(1):15–20.
15. Valkenburg-van den Berg AW, Sprij AJ, Dekker FW, et al. Association between colonization with Group B Streptococcus and preterm delivery: a systematic review. Acta Obstet Gynecol Scand 2009;88(9):958–67.
16. Regan JA, Klebanoff MA, Nugent RP, et al. Colonization with group B streptococci in pregnancy and adverse outcome. VIP Study Group. Am J Obstet Gynecol 1996;174(4):1354–60.
17. Krohn MA, Hillier SL, Baker CJ. Maternal peripartum complications associated with vaginal group B streptococci colonization. J Infect Dis 1999;179(6):1410–5.
18. Gilstrap LC 3rd, Cunningham FG. The bacterial pathogenesis of infection following cesarean section. Obstet Gynecol 1979;53(5):545–9.
19. Martens MG, Kolrud BL, Faro S, et al. Development of wound infection or separation after cesarean delivery. Prospective evaluation of 2,431 cases. J Reprod Med 1995;40(3):171–5.
20. Hill JB, Sheffield JS, McIntire DD, et al. Acute pyelonephritis in pregnancy. Obstet Gynecol 2005;105(1):18–23.
21. Blanco JD, Gibbs RS, Castaneda YS. Bacteremia in obstetrics: clinical course. Obstet Gynecol 1981;58(5):621–5.
22. Cape A, Tuomala RE, Taylor C, et al. Peripartum bacteremia in the era of group B streptococcus prophylaxis. Obstet Gynecol 2013;121(4):812–8.
23. Thomsen AC, Morup L, Hansen KB. Antibiotic elimination of group-B streptococci in urine in prevention of preterm labour. Lancet 1987;1(8533):591–3.
24. Romero R, Oyarzun E, Mazor M, et al. Meta-analysis of the relationship between asymptomatic bacteriuria and preterm delivery/low birth weight. Obstet Gynecol 1989;73(4):576–82.
25. Mittendorf R, Williams MA, Kass EH. Prevention of preterm delivery and low birth weight associated with asymptomatic bacteriuria. Clin Infect Dis 1992;14(4):927–32.
26. Verani JR, McGee L, Schrag SJ. Prevention of perinatal group B streptococcal disease–revised guidelines from CDC, 2010. MMWR Recomm Rep 2010; 59(RR-10):1–36.
27. Aungst M, King J, Steele A, et al. Low colony counts of asymptomatic group B streptococcus bacteriuria: a survey of practice patterns. Am J Perinatol 2004; 21(7):403–7.
28. Anderson BL, Simhan HN, Simons KM, et al. Untreated asymptomatic group B streptococcal bacteriuria early in pregnancy and chorioamnionitis at delivery. Am J Obstet Gynecol 2007;196(6):524.e1–5.
29. Newman TB, Puopolo KM, Wi S, et al. Interpreting complete blood counts soon after birth in newborns at risk for sepsis. Pediatrics 2010;126(5):903–9.
30. Group B streptococcal infections in pregnancy. ACOG Technical Bulletin Number 170–July 1992. Int J Gynaecol Obstet 1993;42(1):55–9.
31. Rouse DJ, Goldenberg RL, Cliver SP, et al. Strategies for the prevention of early-onset neonatal group B streptococcal sepsis: a decision analysis. Obstet Gynecol 1994;83(4):483–94.

32. Prevention of perinatal group B streptococcal disease: a public health perspective. Centers for Disease Control and Prevention. MMWR Recomm Rep 1996; 45(RR-7):1–24.

33. Yancey MK, Schuchat A, Brown LK, et al. The accuracy of late antenatal screening cultures in predicting genital group B streptococcal colonization at delivery. Obstet Gynecol 1996;88(5):811–5.

34. Badri MS, Zawaneh S, Cruz AC, et al. Rectal colonization with group B streptococcus: relation to vaginal colonization of pregnant women. J Infect Dis 1977; 135(2):308–12.

35. Philipson EH, Palermino DA, Robinson A. Enhanced antenatal detection of group B streptococcus colonization. Obstet Gynecol 1995;85(3):437–9.

36. American College of Obstetricians and Gynecologists Committee on Obstetric Practice. ACOG Committee Opinion No. 485: prevention of early-onset group B streptococcal disease in newborns. Obstet Gynecol 2011;117(4):1019–27.

37. Orafu C, Gill P, Nelson K, et al. Perianal versus anorectal specimens: is there a difference in Group B streptococcal detection? Obstet Gynecol 2002;99(6): 1036–9.

38. Jamie WE, Edwards RK, Duff P. Vaginal-perianal compared with vaginal-rectal cultures for identification of group B streptococci. Obstet Gynecol 2004;104(5 Pt 1):1058–61.

39. Price D, Shaw E, Howard M, et al. Self-sampling for group B streptococcus in women 35 to 37 weeks pregnant is accurate and acceptable: a randomized cross-over trial. J Obstet Gynaecol Can 2006;28(12):1083–8.

40. Mercer BM, Taylor MC, Fricke JL, et al. The accuracy and patient preference for self-collected group B Streptococcus cultures. Am J Obstet Gynecol 1995; 173(4):1325–8.

41. Morales WJ, Lim D. Reduction of group B streptococcal maternal and neonatal infections in preterm pregnancies with premature rupture of membranes through a rapid identification test. Am J Obstet Gynecol 1987;157(1):13–6.

42. Honest H, Sharma S, Khan KS. Rapid tests for group B Streptococcus colonization in laboring women: a systematic review. Pediatrics 2006;117(4):1055–66.

43. Goodrich JS, Miller MB. Comparison of culture and 2 real-time polymerase chain reaction assays to detect group B Streptococcus during antepartum screening. Diagn Microbiol Infect Dis 2007;59(1):17–22.

44. Block T, Munson E, Culver A, et al. Comparison of carrot broth- and selective Todd-Hewitt broth-enhanced PCR protocols for real-time detection of Streptococcus agalactiae in prenatal vaginal/anorectal specimens. J Clin Microbiol 2008;46(11):3615–20.

45. Money D, Dobson S, Cole L, et al. An evaluation of a rapid real time polymerase chain reaction assay for detection of group B streptococcus as part of a neonatal group B streptococcus prevention strategy. J Obstet Gynaecol Can 2008;30(9):770–5.

46. Boyer KM, Gotoff SP. Prevention of early-onset neonatal group B streptococcal disease with selective intrapartum chemoprophylaxis. N Engl J Med 1986; 314(26):1665–9.

47. Matorras R, Garcia-Perea A, Madero R, et al. Maternal colonization by group B streptococci and puerperal infection; analysis of intrapartum chemoprophylaxis. Eur J Obstet Gynecol Reprod Biol 1991;38(3):203–7.

48. Tuppurainen N, Hallman M. Prevention of neonatal group B streptococcal disease: intrapartum detection and chemoprophylaxis of heavily colonized parturients. Obstet Gynecol 1989;73(4):583–7.

49. Ohlsson A, Shah VS. Intrapartum antibiotics for known maternal Group B streptococcal colonization. Cochrane Database Syst Rev 2013;(1):CD007467.
50. Van Dyke MK, Phares CR, Lynfield R, et al. Evaluation of universal antenatal screening for group B streptococcus. N Engl J Med 2009;360(25):2626–36.
51. Salkind AR, Cuddy PG, Foxworth JW. The rational clinical examination. Is this patient allergic to penicillin? An evidence-based analysis of the likelihood of penicillin allergy. JAMA 2001;285(19):2498–505.
52. Rimawi RH, Cook PP, Gooch M, et al. The impact of penicillin skin testing on clinical practice and antimicrobial stewardship. J Hosp Med 2013;8(6):341–5.
53. Baker CJ, Byington CL, Polin RA. Policy statement-Recommendations for the prevention of perinatal group B streptococcal (GBS) disease. Pediatrics 2011; 128(3):611–6.
54. Baker CJ, Kasper DL. Correlation of maternal antibody deficiency with susceptibility to neonatal group B streptococcal infection. N Engl J Med 1976;294(14):753–6.
55. Baker CJ, Rench MA, Edwards MS, et al. Immunization of pregnant women with a polysaccharide vaccine of group B streptococcus. N Engl J Med 1988; 319(18):1180–5.
56. Kim SY, Russell LB, Park J, et al. Cost-effectiveness of a potential group B streptococcal vaccine program for pregnant women in South Africa. Vaccine 2014; 32(17):1954–63.
57. Davies HD, Miller MA, Faro S, et al. Multicenter study of a rapid molecular-based assay for the diagnosis of group B Streptococcus colonization in pregnant women. Clin Infect Dis 2004;39(8):1129–35.
58. Gavino M, Wang E. A comparison of a new rapid real-time polymerase chain reaction system to traditional culture in determining group B streptococcus colonization. Am J Obstet Gynecol 2007;197(4):388.e1–4.
59. Young BC, Dodge LE, Gupta M, et al. Evaluation of a rapid, real-time intrapartum group B streptococcus assay. Am J Obstet Gynecol 2011;205(4):372.e1–6.
60. Stoll BJ, Hansen NI, Sanchez PJ, et al. Early onset neonatal sepsis: the burden of group B Streptococcal and E. coli disease continues. Pediatrics 2011;127(5): 817–26.
61. Verani JR, Spina NL, Lynfield R, et al. Early-onset group B streptococcal disease in the United States: potential for further reduction. Obstet Gynecol 2014;123(4): 828–37.
62. Barcaite E, Bartusevicius A, Tameliene R, et al. Prevalence of maternal group B streptococcal colonisation in European countries. Acta Obstet Gynecol Scand 2008;87(3):260–71.
63. Edwards RK, Clark P, Sistrom CL, et al. Intrapartum antibiotic prophylaxis 1: relative effects of recommended antibiotics on gram-negative pathogens. Obstet Gynecol 2002;100(3):534–9.
64. Bizzarro MJ, Dembry LM, Baltimore RS, et al. Changing patterns in neonatal Escherichia coli sepsis and ampicillin resistance in the era of intrapartum antibiotic prophylaxis. Pediatrics 2008;121(4):689–96.
65. Puopolo KM, Eichenwald EC. No change in the incidence of ampicillin-resistant, neonatal, early-onset sepsis over 18 years. Pediatrics 2010;125(5):e1031–8.
66. de Cueto M, Sanchez MJ, Sampedro A, et al. Timing of intrapartum ampicillin and prevention of vertical transmission of group B streptococcus. Obstet Gynecol 1998;91(1):112–4.
67. Turrentine MA, Greisinger AJ, Brown KS, et al. Duration of intrapartum antibiotics for group B streptococcus on the diagnosis of clinical neonatal sepsis. Infect Dis Obstet Gynecol 2013;2013:525878.

68. Fairlie T, Zell ER, Schrag S. Effectiveness of intrapartum antibiotic prophylaxis for prevention of early-onset group B streptococcal disease. Obstet Gynecol 2013;121(3):570–7.
69. Barber EL, Zhao G, Buhimschi IA, et al. Duration of intrapartum prophylaxis and concentration of penicillin G in fetal serum at delivery. Obstet Gynecol 2008; 112(2 Pt 1):265–70.
70. Fiore Mitchell T, Pearlman MD, Chapman RL, et al. Maternal and transplacental pharmacokinetics of cefazolin. Obstet Gynecol 2001;98(6):1075–9.
71. Laiprasert J, Klein K, Mueller BA, et al. Transplacental passage of vancomycin in noninfected term pregnant women. Obstet Gynecol 2007;109(5):1105–10.
72. Bergeron MG, Ke D, Menard C, et al. Rapid detection of group B streptococci in pregnant women at delivery. N Engl J Med 2000;343(3):175–9.
73. Edwards RK, Novak-Weekley SM, Koty PP, et al. Rapid group B streptococci screening using a real-time polymerase chain reaction assay. Obstet Gynecol 2008;111(6):1335–41.
74. El Helali N, Nguyen JC, Ly A, et al. Diagnostic accuracy of a rapid real-time polymerase chain reaction assay for universal intrapartum group B streptococcus screening. Clin Infect Dis 2009;49(3):417–23.
75. Boyer KM, Gadzala CA, Kelly PD, et al. Selective intrapartum chemoprophylaxis of neonatal group B streptococcal early-onset disease. III. Interruption of mother-to-infant transmission. J Infect Dis 1983;148(5):810–6.
76. Lijoi D, Di Capua E, Ferrero S, et al. The efficacy of 2002 CDC guidelines in preventing perinatal group B Streptococcal vertical transmission: a prospective study. Arch Gynecol Obstet 2007;275(5):373–9.
77. Berardi A, Rossi C, Biasini A, et al. Efficacy of intrapartum chemoprophylaxis less than 4 hours duration. J Matern Fetal Neonatal Med 2011;24(4):619–25.

Current Management and Long-term Outcomes Following Chorioamnionitis

Clark T. Johnson, MD, MPH[a,b], Azadeh Farzin, MD[b,c,d],
Irina Burd, MD, PhD[a,b,e],*

KEYWORDS

- Chorioamnionitis • Neonatal sepsis • Endometritis • Fetal infection
- Fetal inflammation • Perinatal infection • Perinatal inflammation • Funisitis

KEY POINTS

- Chorioamnionitis as a process of infection and inflammation that affects the fetus of a gravid mother that can cause significant morbidity.
- Diagnosis of chorioamnionitis is based on a constellation of clinical, laboratory, and/or histopathologic findings, making strict evaluation of the condition challenging.
- Chorioamnionitis is associated with many short-term and long-term neonatal morbidities that cause a significant burden of disease on society.
- With timely diagnosis, broad antibiotic therapy to treat chorioamnionitis, either before delivery or shortly thereafter, can help minimize significant morbidity from the condition.
- Cesarean delivery following chorioamnionitis does not improve perinatal outcomes compared with vaginal delivery.

INTRODUCTION

Chorioamnionitis is defined as the presence of active infection in the amniotic sac that causes inflammatory changes in the mother. Strict diagnosis of chorioamnionitis in the absence of invasive testing is problematic because of a lack of consistency. Multiple signs and symptoms are consistent with chorioamnionitis diagnosed before delivery; diagnostic criteria may vary by provider and institution. As a result, the quantification of the burden of disease of chorioamnionitis is significantly challenging.

The authors have nothing to disclose.
[a] Department of Gynecology and Obstetrics, Johns Hopkins Medical Institutions, 600 North Wolfe Street, Phipps 228, Baltimore, MD 21287, USA; [b] Integrated Research Center for Fetal Medicine, Johns Hopkins Medical Institutions, 600 North Wolfe Street, Phipps 217, Baltimore, MD 21287, USA; [c] Department of Pediatrics, Johns Hopkins Medical Institutions, 1800 Orleans Street, Baltimore, MD 21287, USA; [d] International Center for Maternal & Newborn Health, Johns Hopkins University, 605 North Wolfe Street, Baltimore, MD 21287, USA; [e] Department of Neurology, Johns Hopkins Medical Institutions, 600 North Wolfe Street, Baltimore, MD 21287, USA
* Corresponding author. Integrated Research Center for Fetal Medicine, Department of Gynecology and Obstetrics, 600 North Wolfe Street, Phipps 217, Baltimore, MD 21287.
E-mail address: iburd@jhmi.edu

Chorioamnionitis is traditionally considered to be a polymicrobial process, although there is evidence to suggest that bacterial proliferation may not be the initiating event to cause chorioamnionitis.[1] Notably, many of the associated bacteria tend to colonize amniotic fluid with low virulence.[2] It is unclear what causes these bacteria to transition from colonizers to pathologic contributors and, eventually, to chorioamnionitis.[3] Mycoplasma, in particular, seems to commonly colonize the reproductive tract and can be associated with adverse pregnancy outcomes in certain circumstances.[4]

Maternal complications of chorioamnionitis are primarily short-term, including postpartum hemorrhage, wound infection, and endomyometritis. Pregnancy complications, including preterm labor and delivery, add to the significant burden of disease. Chorioamnionitis in one pregnancy can influence the risk of recurrence in a future pregnancy, although this risk remains low. An obstetric history of delivering a child with group B streptococcus (GBS sepsis) early onset neonatal sepsis is an indication for routine GBS prophylaxis in labor for all future pregnancies.

GBS infections, historically, has been a significant contributor to the burden of disease of chorioamnionitis. Recent policies of screening and prophylaxis in labor have been able to significantly decrease its associated morbidity. Despite aggressive GBS prophylaxis, the rates of intrauterine infection and associated morbidity remain high.

Chorioamnionitis is associated with many short-term and long-term neonatal complications. In cases of preterm birth, the child's risk of cerebral palsy, brain injury, and necrotizing enterocolitis are compounded by the associated increased risk of prematurity.

DISEASE DESCRIPTION

Chorioamnionitis diagnosis varies widely across different institutions and countries, with implications both for treatment protocols and for clinical studies. Fever is commonly used in addition to 2 of the signs from the table to make a diagnosis for study inclusion (**Box 1**).[5] In clinical practice, diagnostic criteria can vary more widely. Clinically, the presence of intrapartum fever warrants attention. With improved clinical outcomes following antibiotic use, the threshold for clinical diagnosis and treatment can be lower than that for inclusion in clinical studies. Fever is the most predictive clinical sign that correlates to associated morbidity, although the presence of other signs is used to make a diagnosis because of the imperfect specificity of fever in the diagnosis of chorioamnionitis.[5]

There does seem to be a relationship between regional anesthesia and fever, which may confound the evaluation of relationships. Increased pyrexia is known to be associated with epidural use.[6] Given the relative importance of fever in the diagnosis of clinical chorioamnionitis, it is not surprising that epidural use and an associated fever

---

Box 1
Signs and symptoms for diagnosis of chorioamnionitis

Fever greater than 100.4°F

Uterine tenderness

Maternal tachycardia

Fetal tachycardia

Purulent amniotic fluid

may have a confounding effect on the clinical diagnosis of chorioamnionitis.[7] It is these types of confounding relationships affecting the clinical diagnosis that make externally consistent diagnosis of chorioamnionitis challenging.

Chorioamnionitis is a global disease, further complicating its assessment.[8] A wide variety of resources across countries can affect the diagnosis and treatment in a particular area, contributing to disparities in the burden of disease. Given the widely variable diagnosis and reporting of the condition and as well as prevalence of confounding factors, such as epidural anesthesia, it becomes challenging to draw firm conclusions about the global epidemiology of clinical chorioamnionitis.

Amniotic fluid sampling and culture can be used in the diagnosis of chorioamnionitis.[9] Unfortunately, because of the invasive nature of the procedure, its widespread use is limited. Culture of the fluid may be an objective assessment of the presence of chorioamnionitis, but clinical utility is limited by the time needed to obtain results as well as the potential colonization of the amniotic fluid without affecting an inflammatory response.

Histopathologic diagnosis is considered to be the gold standard by some, as it avoids some of the subjectivity of clinical diagnosis.[5] Unfortunately, these data may not be available until after delivery, limiting its clinical utility. Clinical scenarios occur whereby a neonate may be discharged from the hospital and clinically well but with a pathologic evaluation of the placenta that demonstrates evidence of chorioamnionitis. Given the high prevalence of histopathologic chorioamnionitis in asymptomatic neonates, this finding may not affect clinical treatment by itself but may be useful in the presence of other clinical signs.[10] This diagnosis may ultimately be of limited importance as an isolated finding in regard to the clinical management of the neonate.[11]

Even within histopathologic diagnosis, multiple criteria exist. The diagnosis of histologic chorioamnionitis is based on the presence of acute changes within the amnion and chorion.[9] Similarly, funisitis involves acute inflammation within the umbilical cord. The diagnosis can be made with the presence of either or both of these findings. Similar to clinical chorioamnionitis, histopathologic diagnosis is challenged by variability among pathologists in reaching a shared diagnosis on a single specimen.[12]

Histopathologic chorioamnionitis has been reported to be in one-fourth of term deliveries.[13] In general, it seems that histologic chorioamnionitis is more common than clinically evident chorioamnionitis, at term or otherwise.[9]

There seems to be a correlation between histologic chorioamnionitis and maternal symptoms, such as fever.[5] Additionally, there seems to be a relationship between severe histopathologic findings and placental abruption.[14] A recent study suggests that acute histopathologic chorioamnionitis at term is usually a result of a noninfectious inflammatory process.[15] The idea that a large number of studies evaluating chorioamnionitis and outcomes are actually based on a diagnosis that is mostly related to a noninfectious process frustrates comprehensive conclusions.

Chorioamnionitis, whether it is diagnosed histopathologically or clinically, leads to the fetal immune response syndrome (FIRS) (**Fig. 1**).[16] Animal studies have shown that preterm and term neonates may have subtle systemic responses to chorioamnionitis but that these responses may lead to significant long-term sequelae.[17–19]

RISK FACTORS

There are multiple known risk factors associated with chorioamnionitis, demonstrated in **Box 2**. Commonly isolated bacteria from cases of chorioamnionitis are outlined in **Box 3**.

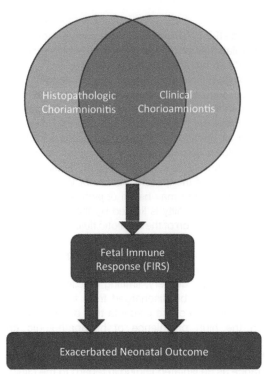

Fig. 1. The relationship between different diagnostic criteria of chorioamnionitis and neonatal outcomes.

Box 2
A list of reported risk factors for the development of chorioamnionitis

Obstetric risk factors for chorioamnionitis

    Prolonged labor

    Prolonged rupture of membranes

    Preterm labor

    Nulliparity

    History of chorioamnionitis in prior pregnancy

    GBS colonization

    Bacterial vaginosis

    Sexually transmitted diseases

    Other genital tract infection

    Meconium stained fluid

    Multiple digital examinations

    Fetal scalp electrodes

    Intrauterine pressure catheters

    Epidural anesthesia

    Tobacco use

    Alcohol use

Box 3
Bacteria that are commonly isolated from and associated with cases of chorioamnionitis

Mycoplasma

Enterobacteriaceae

GBS

Staphylococcus aureus

Gardnerella vaginalis

Neisseria gonorrhoeae

Chlamydia trachomatis

Neonates are at particular risk for sequelae from chorioamnionitis if they are already compromised at the time of delivery. Specific risk factors are listed in **Box 4**.

PREVALENCE/INCIDENCE/MORTALITY RATE

Clinical chorioamnionitis is estimated to affect 1% to 4% of pregnancies worldwide in developed countries.[9] Data are lacking in developing nations but is likely higher than this rate. Maternal bacteremia occurs in 5% to 10 % of women with chorioamnionitis.[9]

The percentage of neonatal deaths attributable to chorioamnionitis is difficult to quantify because the mechanism of injury is caused by significant morbidity, which in turn causes death. The true burden of disease is reflected further when discussing neonatal outcomes.

Similarly, maternal morbidity directly related to chorioamnionitis is difficult to assess. Chorioamnionitis is associated with many obstetric complications that can lead to death, but assessing the precise attribution of chorioamnionitis remains challenging.

GROUP B STREPTOCOCCUS

GBS was the leading cause of neonatal sepsis in the 1970s in the United States (**Fig. 2**).[14] The next decades saw the development of effective treatment of maternal carriers with intravenous (IV) antibiotics, penicillin or otherwise if allergic. Thereafter, the development of standardized screening testing during pregnancy led to universal screening (**Fig. 3**), as recommended by the professional organizations. With the development of consensus guidelines (**Fig. 4**), this led to the dramatic reduction of neonates affected by GBS that is seen today.

Box 4
Underlying neonatal risk factors for potential sequelae following chorioamnionitis

Neonatal risk factors for exacerbation from chorioamnionitis

    Genetic anomalies

    Acidemia

    Delayed antibiotic administration

    Prematurity

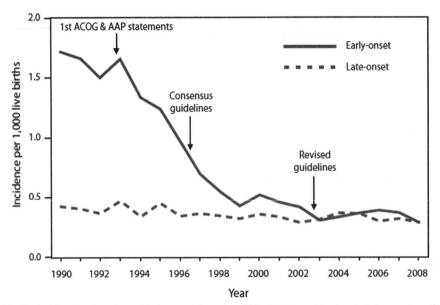

Fig. 2. Incidence of early and late-onset invasive GBS disease: active bacterial core surveillance areas (1990–2008) and activities for prevention of GBS disease. The United States and Western Europe are similar in terms of their prevalence of GBS. AAP, American Academy of Pediatrics; ACOG, American College of Obstetricians and Gynecologists. (*From* Verani JR, McGee L, Schrag SJ. Prevention of perinatal group B streptococcal disease–revised guidelines from CDC, 2010. MMWR Recomm Rep 2010;59(RR-10):3.)

Across different countries, GBS colonization rates vary.[8] However, there is additional evidence that portions of Africa are at similar colonization rates.[8] The Far East has lower reported rates, but this could be because of methodological issues in screening for and reporting GBS colonization.[8] There are significant challenges in assessing GBS prevalence in developing countries and its associated burden of disease to help establish differences in GBS epidemiology in the global arena.[8]

CLINICAL OUTCOMES

Many adverse maternal outcomes are significantly associated with chorioamnionitis (**Box 5**); however, many of these outcomes do not seem to be related to the duration of infection, rather, simply, to its presence.[20] Neonates affected by chorioamnionitis can have significant sequelae (**Box 6**).

Chorioamnionitis has both short-term and long-term complications for the neonate. Cerebral palsy and many of these outcomes are linked to both histology[21–26] and clinical diagnosis.[27–30] One of the challenges in assessing the influence of chorioamnionitis on clinical neonatal outcomes is the different diagnostic criteria used in different studies.

When controlling for major morbidity associated with chorioamnionitis, there does not seem to be an independent relationship between chorioamnionitis and death.[28] With that, any association between chorioamnionitis and death is likely to be mediated through the significant morbidity that it causes.

Chorioamnionitis is clearly associated with an increased risk of a range of morbidities as noted in **Table 1**. Although chorioamnionitis seems to be associated with an

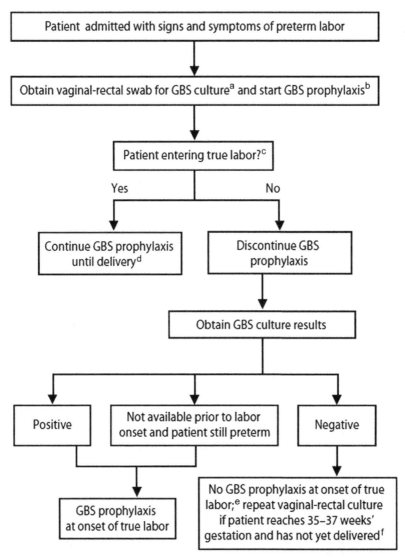

Fig. 3. Algorithm for screening for GBS colonization and use of intrapartum prophylaxis for women with preterm labor (PTL; at <37 weeks and 0 days' gestation). [a] If patient has undergone vaginal-rectal GBS culture within the preceding 5 weeks, the results of that culture should guide management. GBS-colonized women should receive intrapartum antibiotic prophylaxis. No antibiotics are indicated for GBS prophylaxis if a vaginal-rectal screen within 5 weeks was negative. [b] See **Fig. 4** for recommended antibiotic regimens. [c] Patient should be regularly assessed for progression to true labor; if the patient is considered not to be in true labor, discontinue GBS prophylaxis. [d] If GBS culture results become available before delivery and are negative, then discontinue GBS prophylaxis. [e] Unless subsequent GBS culture before delivery is positive. [f] A negative GBS screen is considered valid for 5 weeks. If a patient with a history of PTL is readmitted with signs and symptoms of PTL and had a negative GBS screen greater than 5 weeks prior, she should be rescreened and managed according to this algorithm at that time. (*From* Verani JR, McGee L, Schrag SJ. Prevention of perinatal group B streptococcal disease–revised guidelines from CDC, 2010. MMWR Recomm Rep 2010;59(RR-10):15.)

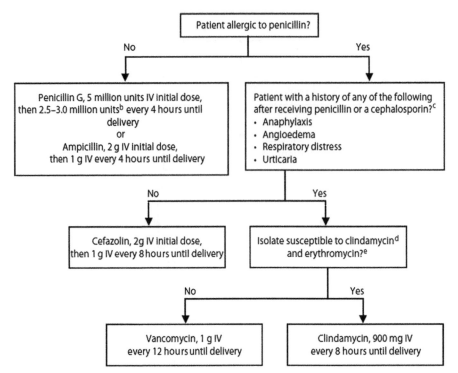

Fig. 4. Recommended regimens for intrapartum antibiotic prophylaxis for prevention of early onset GBS disease. [a] Broader-spectrum agents, including an agent active against GBS, might be necessary for treatment of chorioamnionitis. [b] Doses ranging from 2.5 to 3.0 million units are acceptable for the doses administered every 4 hours following the initial dose. The choice of dose within that range should be guided by which formulations of penicillin G are readily available to reduce the need for pharmacies to specially prepare doses. [c] Penicillin-allergic patients with a history of anaphylaxis, angioedema, respiratory distress, or urticaria following administration of penicillin or a cephalosporin are considered to be at high risk for anaphylaxis and should not receive penicillin, ampicillin, or cefazolin for GBS intrapartum prophylaxis. For penicillin-allergic patients who do not have a history of those reactions, cefazolin is the preferred agent because pharmacologic data suggest it achieves effective intra-amniotic concentrations. Vancomycin and clindamycin should be reserved for penicillin-allergic women at high risk for anaphylaxis. [d] If laboratory facilities are adequate, clindamycin and erythromycin susceptibility testing should be performed on prenatal GBS isolates from penicillin-allergic women at high risk for anaphylaxis. If no susceptibility testing is performed, or the results are not available at the time of labor, vancomycin is the preferred agent for GBS intrapartum prophylaxis for penicillin-allergic women at high risk for anaphylaxis. [e] Resistance to erythromycin is often but not always associated with clindamycin resistance. If an isolate is resistant to erythromycin, it might have inducible resistance to clindamycin, even if it seems susceptible to clindamycin. If a GBS isolate is susceptible to clindamycin and resistant to erythromycin and testing for inducible clindamycin resistance has been performed and is negative (no inducible resistance), then clindamycin can be used for GBS intrapartum prophylaxis instead of vancomycin. (*From* Verani JR, McGee L, Schrag SJ. Prevention of perinatal group B streptococcal disease–revised guidelines from CDC, 2010. MMWR Recomm Rep 2010;59(RR-10):21.)

Box 5
Potential maternal obstetric sequelae associated with chorioamnionitis

Sequelae of chorioamnionitis

Maternal

  Dysfunctional labor

  Increased cesarean delivery risk

  Postpartum hemorrhage

  Blood transfusion

  Postpartum infection

---

increased risk of early onset sepsis as would be expected, there is a decreased risk of late-onset sepsis.[31] It is postulated that the mechanisms of this developed resistance is related to an enhanced immune response, following the inflammatory event at birth that may help to protect the neonate.[31] See **Table 2** for representative studies or meta-analyses evaluating the relationship between chorioamnionitis and selected short-term neonatal outcomes.

MANAGEMENT: PREVENTIVE AND THERAPEUTIC OPTIONS

As discussed, one of the major challenges for the treatment of chorioamnionitis is the imperfect sensitivity and specificity of clinical diagnoses. Previous studies have looked at the use of antibiotics in different populations at high risk for chorioamnionitis with mixed results.[36–38] Currently, it is not recommended to treat patients at risk for chorioamnionitis but rather reserve treatment for when clinical chorioamnionitis is diagnosed, based on a variety of criteria.[39] Excessive use of antibiotics in this setting is associated with inferior neonatal outcomes.[40,41] This finding is consistent with the relationship of prolonged empirical antibiotics administered to neonates being associated with increased morbidity.[42] Antibiotics have been specifically studied in preterm labor with intact membranes without clinical benefit.[43] A specific study evaluating the

---

Box 6
Potential neonatal sequelae associated with chorioamnionitis

Neonatal

Sepsis

Pneumonia

Respiratory distress

Asphyxia

Necrotizing enterocolitis

Intraventricular hemorrhage

Periventricular leukomalacia

Cerebral palsy

Long-term neurodevelopmental delay

Death

Table 1
A summary of representative studies or meta-analyses, evaluating the relationship between chorioamnionitis and selected short-term neonatal outcomes

Neonatal Condition	Study	Study Design	Short-term Outcomes Following Chorioamnionitis		
			Chorioamnionitis Criteria	Sample Size	OR, Adjusted Where Available
Early onset sepsis	Sorashaim et al,[24] 2013	Retrospective cohort (<29 wk)	Histologic	N = 384	5.54 (2.87–10.69)
Late onset sepsis	Strunk et al,[31] 2012	Retrospective cohort (<30 wk)	Histologic	N = 838	0.74 (0.57–0.96)
Peri-intraventricular hemorrhage	Sorashaim et al,[24] 2013	Retrospective cohort (<29 wk)	Histologic	N = 384	1.62 (1.17–2.24)
Periventricular leukomalacia	Garcia-Munoz et al,[28] 2014	Retrospective cohort (VLBW infants)	Clinical	N = 451	24.62 (1.87–324.28)[a]
Necrotizing enterocolitis	Been et al,[32] 2013	Meta-analysis	Clinical, histologic	7 Studies N = 5889	1.24 (1.01–1.52)
Bronchopulmonary dysplasia	Hartling et al,[33] 2012	Meta-analysis	Clinical, histologic	59 Studies N = 15,295	1.89 (1.56–2.3), adjusted for GA 1.58 (1.11–2.24)
Retinopathy of prematurity	Mitra et al,[34] 2014	Meta-analysis	Clinical, histologic	27 Studies N = 10,590	1.33 (1.14–155), adjusted for GA 0.98 (0.77–1.26)

Abbreviations: GA, gestational age; OR, odds ratio; VLBW, very low birth weight (<1500 grams).
[a] Indicates adjusted relative risk (rather than odds ratio).

Table 2
A summary of representative studies or meta-analyses evaluating the relationship between chorioamnionitis and selected short-term neonatal outcomes

Neonatal Condition	Study	Study Design	Chorioamnionitis Criteria	Sample Size	OR (95% CI), Adjusted Where Available
			Long-term Outcomes Following Chorioamnionitis		
Low cognitive score	Pappas et al,[35] 2014	Retrospective cohort	Both histologic and clinical chorioamnionitis	N = 1480	2.00 (1.10–3.64)
Lower language score	Pappas et al,[35] 2014	Retrospective cohort	Both histologic and clinical chorioamnionitis	N = 1480	1.24 (0.83–1.84)
Cerebral palsy	Shatrov et al,[27] 2010	Meta-analysis	Clinical chorioamnionitis	12 Studies	2.41 (1.52–3.84)
Cerebral palsy	Shatrov et al,[27] 2010	Meta-analysis	Histologic chorioamnionitis	8 Studies	1.83 (1.17–2.89)
Neurodevelopmental impairment	Rovira et al,[25] 2011	Prospective cohort	Histologic funisitis	N = 144	4.07 (1.10–15.09)

Abbreviations: CI, confidence interval; OR, odds ratio.

use of empirical metronidazole (Flagyl) and erythromycin did not seem to reduce histologic chorioamnionitis.[44]

ANTIBIOTICS FOR CHORIOAMNIONITIS

IV antibiotics are generally considered to be the preferred treatment of chorioamnionitis where available. Limited studies have suggested the nonsuperiority of specific broad-spectrum regimens, including a combination of ampicillin, gentamycin, and clindamycin, or single-agent piperacillin-tazobactam. Oral options may be considered in areas where IV antibiotics are not available,[45] although there is evidence that oral antibiotic therapy with clindamycin does not seem to significantly reduce the rate of histologic chorioamnionitis.[46] If considered, broad-spectrum regimens including penicillins or cephalosporins and a macrolide antibiotic would be prudent. Administration of appropriate broad spectrum antibiotics can be a particular issue in the global arena as a result of the absence of a variety of antibiotic regimens.

Preterm premature rupture of membranes (PPROM) has been well studied. Management with 2 days of IV antibiotics followed by 5 days of oral antibiotics is associated with increasing the latency between PPROM and delivery.[47,48] Further use of antibiotics beyond this timeline seems to be associated with worse neonatal outcomes without apparent clinical benefit.[39]

The prophylaxis protocol for GBS colonization in labor has been well defined in the United States.[49,50] Consideration for prophylaxis should be considered in the clinical circumstances as noted. Prophylaxis is indicated at the time of induction or labor. Penicillin therapy is preferred because of the very low level of resistance among GBS isolates. In patients with allergy or other contraindication, therapy can be considered as indicated in **Table 3**.

With a diagnosis of chorioamnionitis, delivery should be considered (**Fig. 5**). Although antibiotic therapy with the fetus in utero may temporize the sequelae of chorioamnionitis, extended latency can lead to maternal sepsis with significant morbidity and mortality and is not recommended. Immediate delivery by cesarean is also not indicated. Frequently, nonreassuring fetal status or fetal tachycardia will improve with a combination of antipyretics and antibiotics. Unless contraindicated, induction and trial of labor can and should be undertaken. There is not evidence to suggest that prolongation of a pregnancy complicated by chorioamnionitis leads to worse maternal or neonatal outcomes.

Neonatal management following delivery of chorioamnionitis is to provide secondary prevention against neonatal sepsis and infectious sequelae. Strict surveillance with indicated use of antibiotic and supportive therapy can help avert significant morbidity.

The suggested management for the neonate delivered from a GBS positive mother is shown in **Fig. 4**. This algorithm can be similarly adapted to evaluate neonates following delivery affected by chorioamnionitis to help limit morbidity.

NEONATAL MANAGEMENT

Prompt diagnosis (**Box 7**) of the neonate suspected to be septic should be treated promptly to help avert short- and long-term morbidity. Treatment is composed primarily of broad-spectrum antibiotics, with a penicillin to cover GBS and Listeria monocytogenes and gentamicin to cover Escherichia coli and local gram-negative bacteria. Supportive care should be used, and evaluation for evidence of infection of a particular organ system can guide further antibiotic management (**Fig. 6**).

Table 3
Indications and nonindications for intrapartum antibiotic prophylaxis to prevent early onset GBS disease

Intrapartum GBS Prophylaxis Indicated	Intrapartum GBS Prophylaxis Not Indicated
Previous infant with invasive GBS disease	Colonization with GBS during a previous pregnancy (unless an indication for GBS prophylaxis is present for current pregnancy)
GBS bacteriuria during any trimester of the current pregnancy	
Positive GBS screening culture during current pregnancy[a] (unless a cesarean delivery, is performed before onset of labor on a woman with intact amniotic membranes)	GBS bacteriuria during previous pregnancy (unless another indication for GBS prophylaxis is present for current pregnancy)
Unknown GBS status at the onset of labor (culture not done, incomplete, or results unknown) and any of the following:	Cesarean delivery performed before onset of labor on a woman with intact amniotic membranes, regardless of GBS colonization status or gestational age
• Delivery at <37 wk of gestation[b]	
• Amniotic membrane rupture greater than or equal to 18 h	Negative vaginal and rectal GBS screening culture result in late gestation[a] during the current pregnancy, regardless of intrapartum risk factors
• Intrapartum temperature $\geq$100.4°F ($\geq$38.0°C)[c]	
• Intrapartum NAAT[d,e,f] positive for GBS	

Abbreviation: NAAT, nucleic acid amplification tests.

[a] Intrapartum antibiotic prophylaxis is not indicated in this circumstance if a cesarean delivery is performed before onset of labor on a woman with intact amniotic membranes.

[b] Optimal timing for prenatal GBS screening is at 35 to 37 weeks' gestation.

[c] If amnionitis is suspected, broad-spectrum antibiotic therapy that includes an agent known to be active against GBS should replace GBS prophylaxis.

[d] Recommendations for the use of intrapartum antibiotics for prevention of early onset GBS disease in the setting of threatened preterm delivery are presented in **Fig. 3**.

[e] If amnionitis is suspected, broad-spectrum antibiotic therapy that includes an agent known to be active against GBS should replace GBS prophylaxis.

[f] Nucleic acid amplification tests (NAAT) for GBS is optional and might not be available in all settings. If intrapartum NAAT is negative for GBS but any other intrapartum risk factor (delivery at <37 weeks' gestation, amniotic membrane rupture at $\geq$18 hours, or temperature $\geq$100.4°F [$\geq$38.0°C]) is present, then intrapartum antibiotic prophylaxis is indicated.

From Verani JR, McGee L, Schrag SJ. Prevention of perinatal group B streptococcal disease–revised guidelines from CDC, 2010. MMWR Recomm Rep 2010;59(RR-10):14.

COMPLICATIONS AND CONCERNS

Screening for GBS is imperfect and technically challenging to achieve 100% compliance in any population. Therefore, there remain potential risks of undertreatment in the population and the risk of preventable morbidity. Ultimately, as worldwide efforts to better screen and treat GBS progresses, there will be diminishing returns on investments such as vaccination that might reduce GBS associated morbidity as well as necessary screening and treatment efforts.[51] Studies to develop and implement a vaccine against GBS to be used in the general population have the potential to overcome the limits in the current approach to GBS and prevent morbidity.[4]

Just as screening and treatment of GBS is ultimately imperfect in implementation, there are significant challenges with systematic screening and treatment of chorioamnionitis across the population. The survey of obstetric practice reveals a wide spectrum of clinical criteria for the diagnosis as well as the approach to treatment of chorioamnionitis.[52] Until a uniform diagnostic criterion for chorioamnionitis and women at risk for resultant morbidity can be implemented, challenges in optimizing maternal and neonatal morbidity from chorioamnionitis will be limited. Further efforts to develop better criteria to diagnose and treat chorioamnionitis will help reduce morbidity.[53]

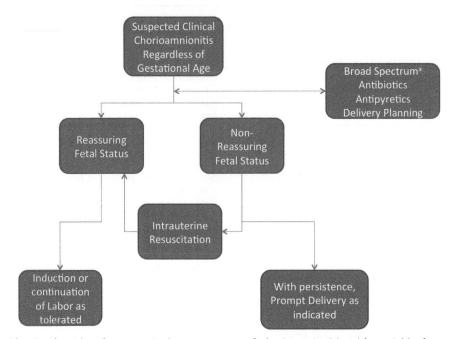

Fig. 5. Algorithm for suggested management of chorioamnionitis with a viable fetus. [a] Broad-spectrum antibiotics consideration may include ampicillin, gentamycin, clindamycin, Flagyl, erythromycin, and piperacillin/tazobactam.

It is the unfortunate reality that chorioamnionitis is a significant risk factor for preterm labor and delivery. Retrospective studies must consider this relationship when evaluating the association with morbidity, as preterm delivery itself is an independent risk factor for many of the morbidities that are associated with chorioamnionitis and, without careful analysis, can overestimate the association of chorioamnionitis with various morbidities.[33,34] A result of this relationship between chorioamnionitis and preterm delivery is a synergistic exacerbation of neonatal morbidity, further incentivizing the importance of diagnosis and treatment of chorioamnionitis.[54]

Betamethasone is well established as an important tool in the prevention of neonatal morbidity resulting from preterm delivery.[55] One might question the utility of immune-suppressing steroids in the setting of chorioamnionitis, out of concern that it might exacerbate infection and neonatal outcomes.[56] A meta-analysis of human studies

---

Box 7
A list of potential diagnostic criteria to evaluate the neonate at risk for sepsis

Neonatal sepsis evaluation

- Blood culture
- Complete blood count/platelets
- White blood cell differential
- Chest radiograph
- Lumbar puncture

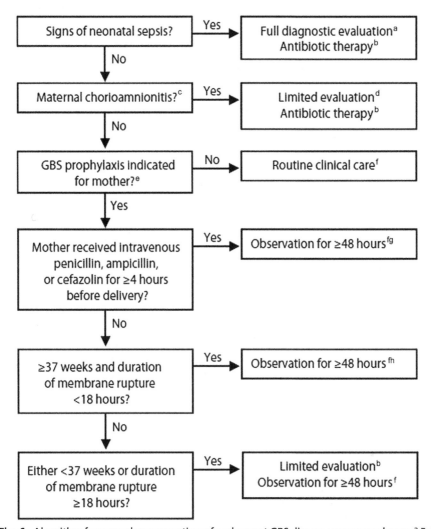

Fig. 6. Algorithm for secondary prevention of early onset GBS disease among newborns. [a] Full diagnostic evaluation includes a blood culture, a complete blood count (CBC) including white blood cell differential and platelet counts, chest radiograph (if respiratory abnormalities are present), and lumbar puncture (if patient is stable enough to tolerate procedure and sepsis is suspected). [b] Antibiotic therapy should be directed toward the most common causes of neonatal sepsis, including IV ampicillin for GBS and coverage for other organisms (including *Escherichia coli* and other gram-negative pathogens) and should take into account local antibiotic resistance patterns. [c] Consultation with obstetric providers is important to determine the level of clinical suspicion for chorioamnionitis. Chorioamnionitis is diagnosed clinically and some of the signs are nonspecific. [d] Limited evaluation includes blood culture (at birth) and CBC with differential and platelets (at birth and/or at 6–12 hours of life). [e] See **Table 3** for indications for intrapartum GBS prophylaxis. [f] If signs of sepsis develop, a full diagnostic evaluation should be conducted and antibiotic therapy initiated. [g] If 37 weeks' gestation or more, observation may occur at home after 24 hours if other discharge criteria have been met, access to medical care is readily available, and a person who is able to comply fully with instructions for home observation will be present. If any of these conditions is not met, the infant should be observed in the hospital for at least 48 hours and until discharge criteria are achieved. [h] Some experts recommend a CBC with differential and platelets at 6 to 12 hours of age. (*From* Verani JR, McGee L, Schrag SJ. Prevention of perinatal group B streptococcal disease–revised guidelines from CDC, 2010. MMWR Recomm Rep 2010;59(RR-10):22; with permission.)

has demonstrated that steroid administration in the setting of prematurity and chorioamnionitis is associated improved neonatal outcomes among a variety of potential morbidities.[57] Chorioamnionitis is not a contraindication to administering steroids to optimize the neonatal outcome of the premature fetus.[55] Efforts should be made to ensure this important intervention is not withheld from preterm pregnancies with chorioamnionitis, lest a significant benefit be withheld from this high-risk population.

Chorioamnionitis is a global disease. Although efforts at improving screening and preventing morbidity have been successful in developed countries with much effort and investment,[58] little progress has been made in the global arena. Efforts to consider international issues in implementing effective screening and treatment strategies will be needed to prevent future morbidity. Efforts to develop a GBS vaccine and implement it in the global arena are examples of successful efforts to bridge this gap.[59] Future efforts to focus on improving screening and the potential for available treatments for chorioamnionitis in a variety of settings will be needed to optimize maternal and neonatal outcomes worldwide.

SUMMARY/DISCUSSION/FUTURE PATHWAYS

Discussion of chorioamnionitis has been focused on clinical or histopathologic chorioamnionitis. Amniotic and intrauterine colonization without evidence of inflammation warrants attention.[3] Within chorioamnionitis, the presence of in utero inflammation seems to significantly exacerbate neonatal outcomes, as opposed to chorioamnionitis without evidence of inflammation.[60] Colonization is seen in amniocentesis samples that grow organisms but without elevated inflammatory markers, such as interleukin-6 (IL-6).[3] Care in interpretation may need to be taken, depending on the colonized organism, specifically some mycoplasma that might have increased pathogenicity and the potential to induce morbidity.[61,62]

A discussion of asymptomatic colonization draws attention to the contrapositive: aseptic amniotic fluid with elevated inflammatory markers (such as IL-6), which may share outcomes as a patient with diagnosed chorioamnionitis.[3] Recent studies have demonstrated this clinical entity, and its management has yet to be established and optimized. Antibiotics would be of limited utility, as the consequences seem to result from inflammation rather than infection; future research will point in this direction to develop effective treatment.

Although much work has been done in inflammatory markers and their association with preterm labor, PPROM, and neonatal compromise, few studies have been able to demonstrate a clinical benefit from their use.[63] One aspect of this challenge is detecting inflammatory markers in a noninvasive manner, to limit risks that may outweigh the potential benefits of the information. In addition, future efforts will have to evaluate treatment modalities, antibiotics, or inflammatory modulating drugs that may help improve outcomes. These studies are urgently needed.

Multiple animal models exist for the study of inflammation and chorioamnionitis.[17–19] Models exist in mice, rats, and rabbits using various infectious organisms and lipopolysaccharide that have developed damage to various areas of the brain (white matter and gray matter) as well as behavioral changes.[17–19] These models, and future models that build on these discoveries, hold much promise for the future studies of chorioamnionitis, inflammation, and their effect on long-term sequelae.

The role of chorioamnionitis in preterm labor is significant, as most preterm deliveries can be attributed to evidence of chorioamnionitis, clinical or pathologic. Future studies evaluating populations with differential risks of preterm labor (eg, multiple gestations, history of prior preterm delivery, and various ethnic minorities) may lead to a better understanding of the contribution of chorioamnionitis to preterm labor and delivery in these populations. As it is likely that the fraction of these deliveries attributed to chorioamnionitis or infection would vary among the different groups, insight may be gained in the further evaluation of these differences.

Efforts at developing a maternal vaccine are well underway. Antepartum treatment seems to confer neonatal protection.[64] The burden of GBS remains, particularly with late-onset GBS sepsis, which is not necessarily treated with current screening regimens.[65] Some of this morbidity may be caused by GBS transmission during breastfeeding.[66] Implementation of a to-be-developed vaccine may even further reduce the horrific morbidity of preventable neonatal sepsis.[65] Studies have evaluated its cost-effectiveness in South Africa and found that implementation of a vaccine would likely be cost-effective and a worthwhile process.[58] In addition, it seems that such a vaccine would be well accepted by an American population.[67] In sum, the vaccination would help reduce preventable morbidity in developed and developing countries.[59,68]

Future directions of management will rely on more specific diagnoses of chorioamnionitis.[53,69] Efforts to develop more rapid evaluation of amniocentesis samples have the potential to provide a rapid and accurate diagnostic test to guide clinical management.[70,71] Optimization of treatment will rely on further delineation of phenotypes of the clinical scenarios, determination and screening for biomarkers as proxies for risk, effective development of significant biochemical pathways, determination of environmental influences on these models, as well as elucidation of the influence of racial and ethnic factors on these pathways.[69] Future interventions will rely on a customization of these factors to best establish an individual's risk in order to implement therapies that are optimized for the individual. Empirical therapy for suspected cases remains the standard of care until that time.

REFERENCES

1. Kim MJ, Romero R, Gervasi MT, et al. Widespread microbial invasion of the chorioamniotic membranes is a consequence and not a cause of intra-amniotic infection. Lab Invest 2009;89(8):924–36.
2. Keski-Nisula L, Kirkinen P, Katila ML, et al. Cesarean delivery. Microbial colonization in amniotic fluid. J Reprod Med 1997;42(2):91–8.
3. Combs CA, Gravett M, Garite TJ, et al, ProteoGenix/Obstetrix Collaborative Research Network. Amniotic fluid infection, inflammation, and colonization in preterm labor with intact membranes. Am J Obstet Gynecol 2014;210(2): 125.e1–15.
4. Schrag SJ, Verani JR. Intrapartum antibiotic prophylaxis for the prevention of perinatal group B streptococcal disease: experience in the United States and implications for a potential group B streptococcal vaccine. Vaccine 2013; 31(Suppl 4):D20–6.
5. Curtin WM, Katzman PJ, Florescue H, et al. Accuracy of signs of clinical chorioamnionitis in the term parturient. J Perinatol 2013;33(6):422–8.
6. Fusi L, Steer PJ, Maresh MJ, et al. Maternal pyrexia associated with the use of epidural analgesia in labour. Lancet 1989;1(8649):1250–2.
7. Abramovici A, Szychowski JM, Biggio JR, et al. Epidural use and clinical chorioamnionitis among women who delivered vaginally. Am J Perinatol 2014. [Epub ahead of print].
8. Le Doare K, Heath PT. An overview of global GBS epidemiology. Vaccine 2013; 31(Suppl 4):D7–12.

9. Tita AT, Andrews WW. Diagnosis and management of clinical chorioamnionitis. Clin Perinatol 2010;37(2):339–54.

10. Hoang D, Charlagorla P, Salafia C, et al. Histologic chorioamnionitis as a consideration in the management of newborns of febrile mothers. J Matern Fetal Neonatal Med 2013;26(8):828–32.

11. Torricelli M, Voltolini C, Conti N, et al. Histologic chorioamnionitis at term: implications for the progress of labor and neonatal wellbeing. J Matern Fetal Neonatal Med 2013;26(2):188–92.

12. Sun CC, Revell VO, Belli AJ, et al. Discrepancy in pathologic diagnosis of placental lesions. Arch Pathol Lab Med 2002;126(6):706–9.

13. Mi Lee S, Romero R, Lee KA, et al. The frequency and risk factors of funisitis and histologic chorioamnionitis in pregnant women at term who delivered after the spontaneous onset of labor. J Matern Fetal Neonatal Med 2011; 24(1):37–42.

14. Nath CA, Ananth CV, Smulian JC, et al, New Jersey-Placental Abruption Study Investigators. Histologic evidence of inflammation and risk of placental abruption. Am J Obstet Gynecol 2007;197(3):319.e1–6.

15. Roberts DJ, Celi AC, Riley LE, et al. Acute histologic chorioamnionitis at term: nearly always noninfectious. PLoS One 2012;7(3):e318–9.

16. Kallapur SG, Presicce P, Rueda CM, et al. Fetal immune response to chorioamnionitis. Semin Reprod Med 2014;32(1):56–67.

17. Burd I, Balakrishnan B, Kannan S. Models of fetal brain injury, intrauterine inflammation, and preterm birth. Am J Reprod Immunol 2012;67(4):287–94.

18. Dada T, Rosenzweig JM, Al Shammary M, et al. Mouse model of intrauterine inflammation: sex-specific differences in long-term neurologic and immune sequelae. Brain Behav Immun 2014;38:142–50.

19. Kannan S, Dai H, Navath RS, et al. Dendrimer-based postnatal therapy for neuroinflammation and cerebral palsy in a rabbit model. Sci Transl Med 2012;4(130): 130–46.

20. Rouse DJ, Landon M, Leveno KJ, et al, National Institute of Child Health And Human Development, Maternal-Fetal Medicine Units Network. The Maternal-Fetal Medicine Units cesarean registry: chorioamnionitis at term and its duration-relationship to outcomes. Am J Obstet Gynecol 2004;191:211–6.

21. Salas AA, Faye-Petersen OM, Sims B, et al. Histological characteristics of the fetal inflammatory response associated with neurodevelopmental impairment and death in extremely preterm infants. J Pediatr 2013;652:7.e1–2.

22. van Vliet EO, de Kieviet JF, van der Voorn JP, et al. Placental pathology and long-term neurodevelopment of very preterm infants. Am J Obstet Gynecol 2012;206(6):489.e1–7.

23. Suppiej A, Franzoi M, Vedovato S, et al. Neurodevelopmental outcome in preterm histological chorioamnionitis. Early Hum Dev 2009;85(3):187–9.

24. Soraisham AS, Trevenen C, Wood S, et al. Histological chorioamnionitis and neurodevelopmental outcome in preterm infants. J Perinatol 2013;33(1):70–5.

25. Rovira N, Alarcon A, Iriondo M, et al. Impact of histological chorioamnionitis, funisitis and clinical chorioamnionitis on neurodevelopmental outcome of preterm infants. Early Hum Dev 2011;87(4):253–7.

26. Perrone S, Toti P, Toti MS, et al. Perinatal outcome and placental histological characteristics: a single-center study. J Matern Fetal Neonatal Med 2012; 25(Suppl 1):110–3.

27. Shatrov JG, Birch SC, Lam LT, et al. Chorioamnionitis and cerebral palsy: a meta-analysis [meta-analysis]. Obstet Gynecol 2010;116(2 Pt 1):387–92.

28. García-Muñoz Rodrigo F, Galán Henríquez GM, Ospina CG. Morbidity and mortality among very-low-birth-weight infants born to mothers with clinical chorioamnionitis. Pediatr Neonatol 2014. http://dx.doi.org/10.1016/j.pedneo.2013.12.007.

29. Alexander JM, Gilstrap LC, Cox SM, et al. Clinical chorioamnionitis and the prognosis for very low birth weight infants. Obstet Gynecol 1998;91(5 Pt 1):725–9.

30. Wu YW, Colford JM Jr. Chorioamnionitis as a risk factor for cerebral palsy: a meta-analysis [meta-analysis]. JAMA 2000;284(11):1417–24.

31. Strunk T, Doherty D, Jacques A, et al. Histologic chorioamnionitis is associated with reduced risk of late-onset sepsis in preterm infants. Pediatrics 2012;129(1):e134–41.

32. Been JV, Lievense S, Zimmermann LJ, et al. Chorioamnionitis as a risk factor for necrotizing enterocolitis: a systematic review and meta-analysis [meta-analysis]. J Pediatr 2013;162(2):236–42.e2.

33. Hartling L, Liang Y, Lacaze-Masmonteil T. Chorioamnionitis as a risk factor for bronchopulmonary dysplasia: a systematic review and meta-analysis [meta-analysis]. Arch Dis Child Fetal Neonatal Ed 2012;97(1):F8–17.

34. Mitra S, Aune D, Speer CP, et al. Chorioamnionitis as a risk factor for retinopathy of prematurity: a systematic review and meta-analysis [meta-analysis]. Neonatology 2014;105(3):189–99.

35. Pappas A, Kendrick DE, Shankaran S, et al. Chorioamnionitis and early childhood outcomes among extremely low-gestational-age neonates. JAMA Pediatr 2014;168(2):137–47.

36. Nabhan AF, Elhelaly A, Elkadi M. Antibiotic prophylaxis in prelabor spontaneous rupture of fetal membranes at or beyond 36 weeks of pregnancy. Int J Gynaecol Obstet 2014;124(1):59–62.

37. Ovalle A, Romero R, Gómez R, et al. Antibiotic administration to patients with preterm labor and intact membranes: is there a beneficial effect in patients with endocervical inflammation? J Matern Fetal Neonatal Med 2006;19(8):453–64.

38. Hutzal CE, Boyle EM, Kenyon SL, et al. Use of antibiotics for the treatment of preterm parturition and prevention of neonatal morbidity: a meta-analysis [meta-analysis]. Am J Obstet Gynecol 2008;199(6):620.e1–8.

39. ACOG (American Congress of Obstetricians and Gynecologists) Committee on Practice Bulletins-Obstetrics. ACOG practice bulletin No. 120: use of prophylactic antibiotics in labor and delivery. Obstet Gynecol 2011;117(6):1472–83.

40. Didier C, Streicher MP, Chognot D, et al. Late-onset neonatal infections: incidences and pathogens in the era of antenatal antibiotics. Eur J Pediatr 2012;171(4):681–7.

41. Bizzarro MJ, Dembry LM, Baltimore RS, et al. Changing patterns in neonatal Escherichia coli sepsis and ampicillin resistance in the era of intrapartum antibiotic prophylaxis. Pediatrics 2008;121(4):689–96.

42. Shah P, Nathan E, Doherty D, et al. Prolonged exposure to antibiotics and its associations in extremely preterm neonates–the Western Australian experience. J Matern Fetal Neonatal Med 2013;26(17):1710–4.

43. Gomez R, Romero R, Nien JK, et al. Antibiotic administration to patients with preterm premature rupture of membranes does not eradicate intra-amniotic infection. J Matern Fetal Neonatal Med 2007;20(2):167–73.

44. Goldenberg RL, Mwatha A, Read JS, et al. The HPTN 024 study: the efficacy of antibiotics to prevent chorioamnionitis and preterm birth. Am J Obstet Gynecol 2006;194(3):650–61.

45. Hopkins L, Smaill F. Antibiotic regimens for management of intraamniotic infection [meta-analysis]. Cochrane Database Syst Rev 2002;(3):CD003254.

46. Ugwumadu A, Reid F, Hay P, et al. Oral clindamycin and histologic chorioamnionitis in women with abnormal vaginal flora. Obstet Gynecol 2006;107(4):863–8.

47. Kenyon SL, Taylor DJ, Tarnow-Mordi W, ORACLE Collaborative Group. Broad-spectrum antibiotics for preterm, prelabour rupture of fetal membranes: the ORACLE I randomised trial. ORACLE Collaborative Group. Lancet 2001; 357(9261):979–88.

48. Kenyon S, Boulvain M, Neilson JP. Antibiotics for preterm rupture of membranes [meta-analysis]. Cochrane Database Syst Rev 2013;(12):CD001058.

49. American ACOG (American Congress of Obstetricians and Gynecologists) Committee on Obstetric Practice. ACOG committee opinion No. 485: prevention of early-onset group B streptococcal disease in newborns. Obstet Gynecol 2011;117(4):1019–27.

50. Verani JR, McGee L, Schrag SJ, Division of Bacterial Diseases, National Center for Immunization and Respiratory Diseases, Centers for Disease Control and Prevention (CDC). Prevention of perinatal group B streptococcal disease–revised guidelines from CDC, 2010. MMWR Morb Mortal Wkly Rep 2010;59(RR-10):1–36.

51. Verani JR, Spina NL, Lynfield R, et al. Early-onset group B streptococcal disease in the united states: potential for further reduction. Obstet Gynecol 2014;123(4): 828–37.

52. Greenberg MB, Anderson BL, Schulkin J, et al. A first look at chorioamnionitis management practice variation among US obstetricians. Infect Dis Obstet Gynecol 2012;2012:628362.

53. Czikk MJ, McCarthy FP, Murphy KE. Chorioamnionitis: from pathogenesis to treatment. Clin Microbiol Infect 2011;17(9):1304–11.

54. Gonçalves LF, Chaiworapongsa T, Romero R. Intrauterine infection and prematurity. Ment Retard Dev Disabil Res Rev 2002;8(1):3–13.

55. ACOG (American Congress of Obstetricians and Gynecologists) Committee on Practice Bulletins-Obstetrics. ACOG practice bulletin No. 127: management of preterm labor. Obstet Gynecol 2012;119(6):1308–17.

56. Joram N, Launay E, Roze JC, et al. Betamethasone worsens chorioamnionitis-related lung development impairment in rabbits. Am J Perinatol 2011;28(8): 605–12.

57. Been JV, Degraeuwe PL, Kramer BW, Zimmermann LJ. Antenatal steroids and neonatal outcome after chorioamnionitis: a meta-analysis [meta-analysis]. BJOG 2011;118(2):113–22.

58. Van Dyke MK, Phares CR, Lynfield R, et al. Evaluation of universal antenatal screening for group B streptococcus. N Engl J Med 2009;360(25):2626–36.

59. Kim SY, Russell LB, Park J, et al. Cost-effectiveness of a potential group B streptococcal vaccine program for pregnant women in South Africa. Vaccine 2014; 32(17):1954–63.

60. Bastek JA, Weber AL, McShea MA, et al. Prenatal inflammation is associated with adverse neonatal outcomes. Am J Obstet Gynecol 2014;210(5):450.e1–10.

61. Horowitz S, Horowitz J, Mazor M, et al. Ureaplasma urealyticum cervical colonization as a marker for pregnancy complications. Int J Gynaecol Obstet 1995; 48(1):15–9.

62. Yoon BH, Romero R, Lim JH, et al. The clinical significance of detecting Ureaplasma urealyticum by the polymerase chain reaction in the amniotic fluid of patients with preterm labor. Am J Obstet Gynecol 2003;189(4):919–24.

63. Genc MR, Ford CE. The clinical use of inflammatory markers during pregnancy. Curr Opin Obstet Gynecol 2010;22(2):116–21.

64. Baker CJ, Carey VJ, Rench MA, et al. Maternal antibody at delivery protects neonates from early onset group B streptococcal disease. J Infect Dis 2014; 209(5):781–8.
65. Burns G, Plumb J. GBS public awareness, advocacy, and prevention–what's working, what's not and why we need a maternal GBS vaccine. Vaccine 2013; 31(Suppl 4):D58–65.
66. Le Doare K, Kampmann B. Breast milk and group B streptococcal infection: vector of transmission or vehicle for protection? Vaccine 2014;32(26):3128–32.
67. Dempsey AF, Pyrzanowski J, Donnelly M, et al. Acceptability of a hypothetical group B strep vaccine among pregnant and recently delivered women. Vaccine 2014;32(21):2463–8.
68. Melin P, Efstratiou A. Group B streptococcal epidemiology and vaccine needs in developed countries. Vaccine 2013;31(Suppl 4):D31–42.
69. Menon R, Taylor RN, Fortunato SJ. Chorioamnionitis–a complex pathophysiologic syndrome. Placenta 2010;31(2):113–20.
70. Romero R, Miranda J, Chaiworapongsa T, et al. A novel molecular microbiologic technique for the rapid diagnosis of microbial invasion of the amniotic cavity and intra-amniotic infection in preterm labor with intact membranes. Am J Reprod Immunol 2014;71(4):330–58.
71. Oh KJ, Lee SE, Jung H, et al. Detection of ureaplasmas by the polymerase chain reaction in the amniotic fluid of patients with cervical insufficiency. J Perinat Med 2010;38(3):261–8.

Prevention and Management of Cesarean Wound Infection

Joseph L. Fitzwater, MD*, Alan T.N. Tita, MD, PhD

KEYWORDS

- Cesarean • Surgical site infections • Wound • Treatment • Management

KEY POINTS

- Postcesarean surgical site infections constitute a major health and economic threat.
- The multiple risk factors for postcesarean wound and other infections include patient characteristics and intrapartum management.
- Optimization of maternal comorbidities, appropriate antibiotic prophylaxis, and good surgical technique may ameliorate the risk of subsequent wound infection.
- Clinical suspicion for wound infection should be raised by fever, wound erythema, incisional drainage, and expanding induration.
- Approaches to wound management combine administration of topical/systemic antibiotics, debridement of necrotic tissue, and application of dressings for a balanced moist environment.
- Necrotizing fasciitis represents a severe, rapidly expanding wound infection, which presents an immediate threat to the life of the patient. Early identification and debridement are critical for survival.

INTRODUCTION

The US Centers for Disease Control and Prevention (CDC) define a surgical site infection (SSI) as an infection at the surgical site within 30 days of the operative procedure, further stratified by depth of infection: superficial incisional, deep incisional, and organ/space (**Box 1**).[1] SSIs place a significant burden on the health care system, representing 21.8% of health care–associated infections, with an estimated 157,500 cases annually in the United States.[2] Prevention of SSIs is a key component of the Joint Commission's quality improvement initiative through the Surgical Care Improvement Project (SCIP). Cataife and colleagues[3] evaluated the impact of SCIP compliance

No conflicts of interest.

Division of Maternal-Fetal Medicine, Department of Obstetrics and Gynecology, University of Alabama at Birmingham, 176F 10270, 619 19th Street South, Birmingham, AL 35249, USA

* Corresponding author.

E-mail address: jfitzwater@uabmc.edu

Obstet Gynecol Clin N Am 41 (2014) 671–689

http://dx.doi.org/10.1016/j.ogc.2014.08.008

obgyn.theclinics.com

Box 1
CDC criteria for surgical site infection

Superficial incisional SSI

Infection occurs within 30 days after the operation and infection involves only skin or subcutaneous tissue of the incision and at least 1 of the following:

1. Purulent drainage, with or without laboratory confirmation, from the superficial incision

2. Organisms isolated from an aseptically obtained culture of fluid or tissue from the superficial incision

3. At least 1 of the following signs or symptoms of infection: pain or tenderness, localized swelling, redness, or heat and superficial incision is deliberately opened by surgeon, unless incision is culture negative

4. Diagnosis of superficial incisional SSI by the surgeon or attending physician

Deep incisional SSI

Infection occurs within 30 days after the operation if no implant is left in place or within 1 year if implant is in place and the infection seems to be related to the operation and infection involves deep soft tissues (eg, fascial and muscle layers) of the incision and at least 1 of the following:

1. Purulent drainage from the deep incision but not from the organ/space component of the surgical site

2. A deep incision spontaneously dehisces or is deliberately opened by a surgeon when the patient has at least 1 of the following signs or symptoms: fever (>38°C), localized pain, or tenderness, unless site is culture negative

3. An abscess or other evidence of infection involving the deep incision is found on direct examination, during reoperation, or by histopathologic or radiologic examination

4. Diagnosis of a deep incisional SSI by a surgeon or attending physician

Organ/space SSI

Infection occurs within 30 days after the operation if no implant is left in place or within 1 year if implant is in place and the infection seems to be related to the operation and infection involves any part of the anatomy (eg, organs or spaces), other than the incision, which was opened or manipulated during an operation and at least 1 of the following:

1. Purulent drainage from a drain that is placed through a stab wound into the organ/space

2. Organisms isolated from an aseptically obtained culture of fluid or tissue in the organ/space

3. An abscess or other evidence of infection involving the organ/space that is found on direct examination, during reoperation, or by histopathologic or radiologic examination

4. Diagnosis of an organ/space SSI by a surgeon or attending physician

Adapted from Mangram AJ, Horan TC, Pearson ML, et al. Guideline for prevention of surgical site infection, 1999. Centers for Disease Control and Prevention (CDC) Hospital Infection Control Practices Advisory Committee. Am J Infect Control 1999;27(2):252.

---

on SSIs in 295 hospital groups and found that compliance with measures, including timely administration of prophylactic antibiotics (ie, within 60 minutes of surgical incision) and use of appropriate antibiotics for a specific procedure, had a large reduction in SSIs. Cesarean delivery, one of the most common major surgical procedures performed worldwide, continues to increase in frequency and is an important contributor to SSIs. In the United States alone, cesareans account for approximately one-third of births or 1.3 million cases annually.[4] Postcesarean SSIs are most commonly superficial or deep wound infections and endomyometritis; less common SSIs include abdominal or pelvic abscesses. Because previous research frequently incorporates endomyometritis with cesarean wound infections as a composite of postcesarean SSIs, there is an overlap in this review regarding their risks and management of wound infections and other SSIs. Whenever possible, information that is specific to postcesarean wound infections is also discussed.

EPIDEMIOLOGY
Prevalence and Morbidity

Postcesarean SSIs within 30 days of delivery have a reported incidence from about 3.7% to 9.8% internationally.[5–11] The variation in incidence reflects differences in risk factors, including antibiotic prophylaxis practices and duration of ascertainment, because most cases of wound infection present after discharge from the delivery admission. One study reported an SSI increase from 1.8% at initial discharge to 8.9% at 30 days postpartum.[5] The temporal risk of postcesarean SSIs has decreased significantly from historical risks exceeding 25% to 50%,[12] likely because of ongoing improvements in antibiotic prophylaxis, sterile procedures, and other practices. Although the maternal mortality ratio associated with cesarean deliveries has historically been low at 5.8/100,000, puerperal infections, including postcesarean infections, are a significant risk factor for maternal morbidity.[13] Bodelon and colleagues[14] reviewed 896 peripartum hysterectomies and discovered that postpartum infection is a serious risk factor, with an odds ratio (OR) of 2.5 (95% confidence interval [CI] 1.5–4.1) during birth admission, and 20.8 (95% CI 8.6–50.2) with readmission. In addition, the economic impact of infections is tremendous, with a doubling of length of stay, with an SSI.[15] In 1 study,[16] the additional costs of a wound infection and endometritis were estimated to be approximately $3700 and $4000, respectively (in 2008 dollars).

Risk Factors for Postcesarean Surgical Site Infection

A myriad of risk factors have been reported for postcesarean-related SSIs, including antepartum factors: low socioeconomic status, limited prenatal care, obesity, tobacco use, diabetes mellitus (pregestational and gestational), significant maternal comorbidities (American Society of Anesthesiologists class of 3 or more), hypertensive disorders, multiple gestations, and corticosteroid administration; intrapartum factors: unscheduled or nonelective cesarean, length of labor, length of rupture of membranes, number of vaginal examinations, internal fetal monitors, chorioamnionitis, duration of operation, absence of antibiotic prophylaxis, management by teaching service, and wound length; and postpartum factors: subcutaneous drains, anemia, and postoperative hematoma (**Table 1**).[5–12,17–27] Although some of these studies evaluated wound infections specifically, it is frequently incorporated in a composite outcome, including other infectious complications (postcesarean SSIs) or with noninfectious complications like wound breakdown as composite wound morbidity. Thus, some of these associations may overestimate or underestimate the specific relationship with wound infections. In addition, reported associations vary depending on the covariates included in adjusted models. Selected risk factors are discussed.

Obesity

A frequent specter in medicine, expanding waistlines are trending upward. Because obesity brings multiple comorbidities and complications, it is not surprising that it has been the subject of intense review. Opøien reported in a prospective cohort of 326 cesarean deliveries a diagnosis of SSI in 29 (8.9%) patients identifying independent risks in body mass index (BMI, calculated as weight in kilograms divided by

Table 1
Risk factors for postcesarean SSIs

Risk Factor	One Decimal Place[a]	References
Antepartum Factors		
Limited prenatal care	3.4	[24]
Obesity	1.1–3.7	[5,6,9–11,17,18]
Tobacco use	2.9–5.32	[19,20]
Diabetes mellitus	1.4–2.5	[7,9,27]
Maternal ASA class ≥3	5.3	[10]
Hypertensive disorders	1.7–2.3	[9,10]
Multiple gestations	1.6	[9]
Corticosteroid administration	3.11	[21]
Intrapartum Factors		
Nonelective vs elective	1.3–2.5	[9,18]
Labor	1.3–4.01	[12,24]
Rupture of membranes	1.3–2.61	[9,12,24]
Vaginal examinations	2.19	[12]
Chorioamnionitis	5.62–10.6	[10,20]
Duration of operation	1.01–2.4	[5,24]
Absence of antibiotic prophylaxis	1.7	[24]
Teaching service	2.7	[6]
Wound length (>166 mm)	4.89	[21]
Postpartum Factors		
Subcutaneous drains	2.24	[19]
Increased blood loss	1.3	[10]
Postoperative hematoma	11.6	[6]

[a] Risk ratio or odds ratio where appropriate.

the square of height in meters) greater than 30 (OR 2.8, 95% CI 1.3–6.2).[5] A prospective study measuring the subcutaneous depth in 140 women, found a significant risk factor in subcutaneous tissue thickness (relative risk [RR] 2.8, 1.3–5.9). The 11 infected patients in this study had an average thickness of 4.1 cm, with a BMI of 49.7.[17] Myles and colleagues[18] evaluated obesity in elective and nonelective cesarean deliveries, finding it to be an independent risk factor for postoperative infection in both cases. A study examining 19,416 cesarean deliveries from Israel[9] showed an increased risk of wound infection from obesity (OR 2.2, 95% CI 1.6–3.1), but obesity with diabetes further increased this risk to an OR of 9.3 (95% CI 4.5–19.2). Wloch and colleagues[11] further substratified BMI risk and showed an increasing OR of postcesarean infection, with increments of BMI as follows: BMI 25 to 30 (OR 1.6, 95% CI 1.2–2.2), 30 to 35 (OR 2.4, 95% CI 1.7–3.4), and greater than 35 (OR 3.7, 95% CI 2.6–5.2). In the same vein, Tran and colleagues[10] identified multiple independent risk factors for SSI, and their evaluation of BMI found an OR of 2.0 for every 5-unit increment (95% CI 1.3–3.0).

Diabetes mellitus

Diabetes mellitus is a long-recognized comorbidity associated with postoperative wound complication in the surgical literature.[28–30] Poorly controlled diabetes results in advanced glycosylation end products, with impairment of the host immune response and decreased reepithelialization of wounds. Over time, diabetes can result in neuropathy and then to unnoticed, repetitive trauma. Microvascular disease results in tissue ischemia and inadequate transportation of oxygen.[28,29]

A retrospective study of 75,947 deliveries determined an SSI rate of 3.97%, with a significant association with gestational diabetes mellitus (OR 1.5, 95% CI not given) among other factors.[7] A study comparing 185 pregestational diabetic patients and 174 nondiabetic patients[27] found a significant association of wound complications with diabetes mellitus. After adjusting for BMI, length of surgery, and previous cesarean delivery, the OR was 2.5 (95% CI 1.1–5.5).

Intrapartum factors

Several intrapartum factors and interventions may result in increased intrapartum and postoperative wound complications, whereas other factors may afford protection. Unscheduled cesareans (after labor, induction, or undertaken for other reasons) constitute a broad subcategory of cesarean delivery at increased risk for postcesarean SSIs. Emmons and colleagues[22] reviewed 60 wound infections after cesarean delivery in a case-control study. They found significant differences in the length of the first stage of labor as well as rupture of membranes, number of vaginal examinations, length of time with internal fetal monitors in place, second stage of labor, and suprafascial drains. Pelle and colleagues[26] had similar findings, with increased wound infection with nonelective operations, rupture of membranes, internal monitors, and obesity. Killian and colleagues[24] showed an increased risk of SSI with absence of antibiotic prophylaxis (OR 2.6, 95% CI 1.5–4.6) and a significant decrease in infection with antibiotic administration regardless of labor or membrane rupture status. In addition to obesity, Myles and colleagues[18] determined that intrapartum factors associated with postoperative infection included labor length and number of vaginal examinations. A case-control study of 1605 cesarean deliveries by Olsen and colleagues[6] identified independent risk factors for SSI in addition to obesity as operation by a teaching service (OR 2.7, 95% CI 1.4–5.2) and development of subcutaneous hematoma (OR 11.6, 95% CI 4.1–33.2). Charrier and colleagues[8] examined a low-risk cohort of women who underwent cesarean delivery and found a significant association between length of membrane rupture and SSI. Although Alexander and colleagues[31] identified a statistically significant increased rate of chorioamnionitis and length of labor, their comparison of almost 12,000 primary cesarean deliveries suggested no difference between the first and second stage of labor in endometritis or wound complications.

Corticosteroids

Patients' medications may interfere with wound healing, such as those on chronic corticosteroids. An unintended side effect of suppressing the immune system is a direct impairment of the inflammatory phase of wound closure. As a result, there is decreased fibrogenesis, macrophage response, and angiogenesis.[28,29] This situation may lead to delayed closure, wound breakdown, and chronic wound formation and infection. In 1 study of 212 consecutive elective cesarean deliveries, wound length greater than 166 mm (OR 4.9, 95% CI 2.4–10.1) and corticosteroid administration (OR 3.1, 95% CI 1.4–7.0) were independently associated with a composite wound morbidity.[21]

PREVENTION OF WOUND INFECTION

The prevention of postcesarean wound infections focuses on limiting the modifiable risk factors.

Labor Management

Based on the close association between cesarean wound infection and labor characteristics such as length of labor, length of ruptured membranes, and intrapartum infection, it is logical to find ways to reduce postoperative complications. Therefore, physician interventions should be carefully considered, with the recognition of potential unintended consequences. In part with this factor in mind, there is an overarching effort to provide labor management guidelines that promote vaginal deliveries and avoid unnecessary cesarean deliveries, because of their consequences, including the more than 5 to 10 times increase in the risk of SSIs.[32]

Management of Comorbidities

An effective preventative for obese women specifically is subcutaneous tissue closure at cesarean. One study randomized 68 women with up to 2 cm subcutaneous tissue and 91 with greater than 2 cm to closure. Although there was no difference in the first group, the second had a significant decrease in the primary outcome of wound disruption, including those caused by infections (27.2% in no closure vs 10.6% in closure).[33] Chelmow and colleagues[34] performed a meta-analysis of 6 randomized controlled trials for subcutaneous closure at cesarean delivery, finding a 34% decrease in risk of wound disruption in patients with a depth greater than 2 cm (number needed to treat 16.2). Closure of subcutaneous tissue decreases the wound disruption rate, although this may primarily be the decrease of wound seromas and not infection.

Overall, the literature is lacking adequate studies for recommendations specific to the management of obese women undergoing cesarean delivery. The optimal skin incision (including transverse vs vertical) remains unclear.[19,25,35] However, drains are not effective and are not recommended.[36,37]

For diabetic patients, postoperative glycemic control is paramount to prevent SSIs. Ideally, pregestational diabetics present for obstetric care early in gestation and maintain compliance with tight glycemic control.

Managing patients on immunosuppressants like corticosteroids can be complicated. Ideally, corticosteroids should be discontinued or tapered before delivery, but usually, the patient's comorbidity precludes these options. Some studies have suggested a benefit from vitamin A in reversing the deleterious effects of corticosteroids. Dosages between 10,000 IU/d and 25,000 IU/d are suggested to bolster wound healing.[28–30,38] An animal model evaluating the interaction of corticosteroids with retinoid therapy[39] showed a suppression of collagen synthesis and growth factors with corticosteroids alone, which was partially reversed by retinoids.

Maintenance of intraoperative normothermia in general surgery has become standard practice because of the risks of SSI with hypothermia. Therefore, this treatment has been recommended for obstetric patients as well.[35] The obstetric-specific data are limited. A case-control study of 18 patients of wound infection found no difference in immediate postoperative temperature with controls.[40]

Antibiotic Prophylaxis

Antibiotic prophylaxis is one of the most important interventions to reduce postcesarean wound and other SSIs. Over the last several decades, there has been an evaluation of antibiotic administration for cesarean prophylaxis, involving the candidates for prophylaxis (elective or nonelective), timing of administration, and choice of antibiotic. Prophylactic antibiotic administration with cesarean delivery is integral in reducing puerperal infection, because cesarean alone increases this risk by 5-fold to 20-fold compared with vaginal delivery.[12] When administering an antibiotic for prophylaxis, the American College of Obstetricians and Gynecologists (ACOG) recommends a narrow-spectrum agent (eg, cefazolin) able to reach therapeutic levels against the most likely pathogens at time of microbial exposure. Caution should be taken to avoid excessively broad coverage, because this can promote bacterial resistance.[41]

A recent review[42] presented the historical and current antibiotic prophylaxis recommendations. Initial concern regarding administration of antibiotics before cord clamp, leading to untoward neonatal effects, including selecting bacterial resistance and masking neonatal sepsis, has been superseded by information suggesting reduction in postcesarean SSIs without evidence of such untoward effects. Furthermore, meta-analyses have helped determine that there is maternal benefit associated with antibiotic prophylaxis for both elective as well as nonelective cesareans, and placebos are no longer ethical in trials of antibiotic prophylaxis with cesarean delivery.[43] Neonatal effects should be evaluated further. The most recent randomized trials evaluating antibiotic administration within 60 minutes before incision have not shown an impact on neonatal sepsis but were not powered for this evaluation.[42] Although a few clinical trials show a decrease in total infection with extended-spectrum regimens (eg, addition of azithromycin or metronidazole to the standard regimen), they have not been adopted widely and remain investigational. A rationale for inclusion of broad-spectrum antibiotics is that first-generation cephalosporins do not cover for anaerobes or *Ureaplasma*, which are commonly identified in wound infections.[42] ACOG does not endorse its routine use and notes that the findings are comparable with the reduction in infection with the change to antibiotic administration before incision.[41] Therefore, a single-dose first-generation cephalosporin, ampicillin, or clindamycin, with an aminoglycoside for patients with a life-threatening drug allergy to penicillins, are the recommended first-choice regimens for antibiotic prophylaxis for cesarean delivery. Consideration may be given to adding vancomycin for patients who are known positive for methicillin-resistant *Staphylococcus aureus* (MRSA), but they do not recommend routine screening (**Box 2**). A Cochrane review[44] in 2010 reported a similar efficacy between penicillins and cephalosporins.

A dose of 1 g of cefazolin is sufficient, but an augmented dose can be considered in patients with a higher BMI.[41] Pevzner and colleagues[45] sampled cefazolin concentrations after administration of 2 g in the adipose tissue, serum, and myometrium at time of cesarean. All of the specimens showed therapeutic levels against gram-positive cocci, but minimum inhibitory concentration (MIC) was not achieved for gram-negative rods in many obese and extremely obese patients' adipose samples. This

---

Box 2
Antibiotic choices for cesarean prophylaxis

Single dose within 60 minutes of incision:

Cephalosporin (preferably first-generation because of cost and equivalent efficacy with later generations) or

Ampicillin (shorter half-life than cefazolin)

If penicillin allergic:

   Clindamycin + aminoglycoside

Consider adding vancomycin if known MRSA carrier.

Addition of azithromycin for adjunctive therapy is under investigation.

Data from American College of Obstetricians and Gynecologists. ACOG practice bulletin No. 120: use of prophylactic antibiotics in labor and delivery. Obstet Gynecol 2011;117(6):1472–83.

finding raises the concern that the standard doses of antibiotics are insufficient for obese patients.

Antiseptic Preparation

Optimal skin preparation for cesarean delivery has not been well defined. The Cochrane and other reviews on this topic[46,47] reflect the insufficient literature, indicating that there is not enough evidence to recommend one preparation (see later discussion) over the other. Nevertheless, a shift has begun toward chlorhexadine-alcohol and away from providone-iodine. In 1 trial,[48] chlorhexadine-alcohol was compared with providone-iodine preparatory scrub. A total of 849 patients were randomized to one of the 2 preparations, and SSI was significantly lower in the chlorhexadine group (RR 0.59, 95% CI 0.41–0.85). Although this treatment was protective against superficial and deep incisional infections, it did not provide a benefit against organ-space infections. A Cochrane meta-analysis by Haas and colleagues[49] examined 5 trials evaluating vaginal preparation compared with no vaginal preparation before cesarean delivery. Preparation with vaginal providone-iodine immediately before cesarean was beneficial in patients both with intact and with ruptured membranes.

Operative Technique

Although intrapartum risk factors can be modified with varying success, there are several operative surgical steps that may decrease the rate of SSI. The CDC guideline from 1999 provides a list of key areas that affect SSI during the operation (**Box 3**). In addition, Duff[50] summarized key techniques to preventing cesarean complications. Those techniques pertaining to infection prevention are listed in **Box 4**.

Two intraoperative techniques to prevent SSI that are not recommended include supplemental oxygen and cervical dilation. Randomized controlled trials evaluating the administration of supplemental oxygen during delivery and for 2 hours afterward have not shown a benefit. In addition, randomized controlled trials have evaluated

---

Box 3
CDC key factors for prevention of SSIs

Patient Factors	Operative Factors
Age	Duration of surgical scrub
Nutritional status	Skin antisepsis
Diabetes	Preoperative shaving
Smoking	Preoperative skin prep
Obesity	Duration of operation
Concurrent infections	Antimicrobial prophylaxis
Colonization with microorganisms	Operating room ventilation
Altered immune response	Inadequate sterilization of instruments
Length of preoperative stay	Foreign material in the surgical site
	Surgical drains
	Surgical technique
	Poor hemostasis
	Failure to obliterate dead space
	Tissue trauma

Adapted from Mangram AJ, Horan TC, Pearson ML, et al. Guideline for prevention of surgical site infection, 1999. Centers for Disease Control and Prevention (CDC) Hospital Infection Control Practices Advisory Committee. Am J Infect Control 1999;27(2):256.

Box 4
Recommended operative techniques

- Clip the hair at the surgical site just before making the incision

- Cleanse the skin with a chlorhexidine solution rather than a povidone-iodine solution

- Administer broad-spectrum systemic antibiotic prophylaxis before the surgical incision rather than after the neonate's umbilical cord is clamped

- Remove the placenta by traction on the umbilical cord rather than by manual extraction

- In women whose subcutaneous tissue is greater than 2 cm in thickness, close the layer with a running suture

Data from Duff P. A simple checklist for preventing major complications associated with cesarean delivery. Obstet Gynecol 2010;116(6):1393–6.

---

the dilation of the cervix after removal of the placenta to allow better evacuation of the uterus, and no benefit was seen.[46]

As mentioned earlier, subcutaneous drains have been ineffective as well. A follow-up trial to subcutaneous closure added subcutaneous drains for women with a subcutaneous depth of 4 cm or deeper, but this did not improve composite wound morbidity (RR 1.3, 95% CI 0.8–2.1) or affect individual wound complication rates, including infection rates.[51] Alanis and colleagues[19] found subcutaneous drains to be an independent risk factor for wound complications in the massively obese patient (BMI $\geq$50), with an OR of 2.3 (95% CI 1.2–4.4). Two meta-analyses regarding prophylactic wound drain placement at time of cesarean delivery concluded that this did not prevent wound disruption and was not recommended.[36,37]

Dressing

There are a multitude of dressings available for a primary wound, ranging from plain gauze to advanced materials like permeable films and antimicrobial dressings. Walter and colleagues[52] examined 16 controlled trials on meta-analysis and did not find one dressing type superior to another or significant differences in patient pain or scarring. A retrospective study[53] examined the effectiveness of silver-impregnated dressings with traditional dressings. There was no significant difference in postoperative wound visits or culture-proven infections. Another recent innovation is the expansion of negative pressure wound therapy to use on the closed incision. These treatments include containerless pressure wound systems like PICO (Smith & Nephew Medical Ltd, Hull, United Kingdom) and Prevena (KCI, Inc, San Antonio, TX, USA). Hudson and colleagues[54] reported that the proposed benefits include decreased wound drainage, reduced seromas/hematomas, and reduced infection/dehiscence in high-risk patients. Although there is not a container, the dressing is designed for high evaporation and can be worn up to 7 days. A meta-analysis of 5 trials by Webster and colleagues[55] did not find a clear benefit in this system over standard therapy, especially in light of the cost. An abstract by Gibbs and colleagues[56] examined the Prevena negative pressure wound therapy against traditional dressings on closed incisions. The initial complication rate was higher in the negative pressure wound therapy arm but appeared to be equivalent when controlling for comorbidities (OR 1.7, 95% CI 0.8–3.8). Therefore, routine use of these systems is discouraged until more compelling data are available. Toon and colleagues[57,58] reviewed trials regarding early dressing removal (before 48 hours) as well as early bathing and reported that the data were limited, but neither appeared harmful.

DIAGNOSIS OF WOUND INFECTIONS
Pathophysiology of Wounds

Acute injuries progress through 3 phases: inflammatory, proliferative, and maturation/remodeling, as shown in (**Box 5**). The inflammatory state is characterized clinically by warmth, swelling, erythema, pain, and loss of function.[59] During this time, hemostasis sets in during the first few minutes, followed by a host immune response over the next 3 to 5 days.[28] The development of fibrin clot acts as a latticework for leukocytes, and the platelets release chemotactic factors. The neutrophils and monocytes arrive to kill bacteria and phagocytize damaged matrix proteins.[60] The macrophages release growth factors to stimulate healing. Proliferation sets in over 4 to 14 days after injury.[28] During this phase, adjacent epidermal keratinocytes move into the wound for reepithelialization. Granulation tissue develops, and angiogenesis is promoted.[60] The epithelial cells adjacent to the wound move inward and fibroblasts migrate into the wound. This process is promoted by a moist environment.[28] In the maturation or remodeling phase, type I collagen steadily begins to replace type III collagen, with tensile strength returning to around 80% of the original around a year after the initial insult.[59] Pathologic disorders such as infections disrupt the transitioning between these phases, resulting in a repetitive cycle of injury and delayed healing.[60]

Microbiology

Evaluation for possible pathogens has been performed in the past to hone the optimal therapy. Studies show that postcesarean SSIs are polymicrobial, with atypical organisms such as *Ureaplasma* involved in many. Roberts and colleagues[61] obtained culture swabs and aspirates from abdominal wounds on 65 patients. Their rate of culture-positive wounds was 72%. The most common isolates were as follows: *Ureaplasma* (62%), coagulase-negative staphylococci (32%), *Enterococcus faecalis* (28%), *Mycoplasma* (21%), anaerobes (15%), gram-negative rods (9%), *Staphyloccocus aureus*

Box 5
Wound timeline

Phases

Inflammatory (*hours to days*)

   Clinical signs of warmth, swelling, erythema, pain, and loss of function

   Hemostasis, platelets release chemotactic factors

   Neutrophils, monocytes, and macrophages arrive at wound bed and phagocytize bacteria and debris

Proliferative (*days to weeks*)

   Epidermal keratinocytes reepithelialize the wound bed

   Development of granulation tissue

   Angiogenesis

Maturation/Remodeling (*up to a year*)

   Type III collagen replaced by type I collagen

   Wound contraction

   Wound regains up about 80% of its original tensile strength

Data from Li J, Chen J, Kirsner R. Pathophysiology of acute wound healing. Clin Dermatol 2007;25(1):9–18.

(6%), and group B *Streptococcus* (2%) (**Table 2**). Another study[62] evaluated cultures from the intact chorioamnion at time of cesarean on 575 patients. *Ureaplasma* was present in 10% of all cultures, and significantly it was present in 28% of patients who developed endometritis.

Clinical Diagnosis

Daily evaluation of the cesarean incision is important during the postoperative period, especially in patients who are at greater risk for wound complications. Warning signs include fever, tenderness, expanding erythema around the wound edges, copious wound drainage (serosanguinous or purulent), and induration. The clinical picture may be clouded by treatment of a concurrent infection such as endomyometritis, because the patient already is on antibiotics.[63] As reflected in previous studies, most wound complications are not identified until after discharge, around days 4 to 7.[5,63] Therefore, patients should be given clear-cut instructions regarding these signs and encouraged to present for evaluation with such concerns.

MANAGEMENT OF WOUND INFECTIONS

Antibiotics, wound exploration, and debridement as indicated are the mainstays of the medical care of postcesarean wound infections.

Antibiotics

Despite the best intentions, cesarean incisions become infected and may require readmission, with operative evaluation. Because the initial appearance of wounds may be deceptive, early intervention is important to circumvent severe complications. When there is evidence of a pelvic infection after a cesarean delivery, empirical coverage should be broad spectrum, including anaerobic coverage. This strategy accounts for most pathogens associated with cesarean infections. Acceptable regimens include clindamycin with an aminoglycoside or aztreonam, extended-spectrum penicillins (eg, piperacillin/tazobactam), and carbapenems. Ampicillin

Table 2 Common cesarean wound pathogens (including frequency encountered)	
Ureaplasma species	62%
Coagulase-negative staphylococci	32%
Enterococcus faecalis	28%
Mycoplasma species	21%
Anaerobes *Propionibacterium acnes* *Streptococcus intermedius* *Clostridium subterminale* *Peptostreptococcus prevotii* *Bacteroides distasonis*	15%
Gram-negative rods *Acinetobacter calcoaceticus* *Serratia marsescens* *Pseudomonas aeruginosa*	9%
Staphyloccocus aureus	6%
Group B *Streptococcus*	2%

Adapted from Roberts S, Maccato M, Faro S, et al. The microbiology of post-cesarean wound morbidity. Obstet Gynecol 1993;81(3):384.

may be added to the regimen with clindamycin and an aminoglycoside for better coverage of enterococcus. Vancomycin should be added to other regimens when there is suspicion for S aureus.[64] Parenteral antibiotics should be discontinued once cellulitis or systemic infection have resolved, because they have poor wound penetration, and frequently, they are unnecessary for infection restricted to the incision.[29]

Wound Debridement

Conservative therapy with antibiotics alone may be attempted if a wound infection seems superficial and without purulence (cellulitis). If the wound has purulent drainage or is concerning for a deep incisional SSI, further wound exploration and debridement are the most important actions. When evaluating a wound, it is helpful to evaluate the components to address for optimal healing: tissue, infection, moisture, and edge of wound.[65] Sharp debridement should remove the wound of all necrotic tissue and debris.[29] In theory, this debris obstructs the migration of healthy tissue and serves as a nidus for infection. An evaluation of debridement techniques does not show that one is superior to the others, because of an inability to compare trials.[66] Sterile conditions may be unrealistic, but less than 10^5 bacterial load per gram of tissue is associated with 94% wound healing.[29] When bacterial overgrowth is suspected to be the source of poor wound healing, topical antiseptic agents may be placed on the wound. These agents include silvadene, bacitracin, polymyxin, and silver nitrate.[29]

In cases of fascial dehiscence, the debridement required to identify healthy tissue may preclude fascial closure. When faced with this choice, placement of mesh can be considered or the fascia allowed to heal by secondary intention. McNeeley and colleagues[67] reported the use of synthetic mesh closure in 18 patients with wound infection for fascial dehiscence. Although 3 patients returned to the operating room for reoperation (1 for debridement and the other 2 for fascial revision), most of the patients healed by secondary intention and without complications.

Necrotizing Fasciitis

Necrotizing fasciitis is a severe disruption of a surgical wound characterized by a rapidly expanding gangrenous infection along the fascial planes involving the deeper skin and subcutaneous tissues. Diabetes, cancer, and other immune-compromised states are risk factors. Goepfert and colleagues[68] described 9 cases over a 7-year period. Although 1 patient had metastatic breast cancer, the patients were healthy overall, without anticipated comorbidities like diabetes mellitus or peripheral vascular disease. The mean time from cesarean delivery to diagnosis was 10 days. Two of the patients died: one from complications of malignancy and the other from sepsis. Early and aggressive surgical debridement is critical. Gallup and Meguiar[69] reviewed the management of necrotizing fasciitis. This is a life-threatening condition, with mortality as high as 50%. Signs for diagnosis include a bluish-brown skin discoloration and sensory deficits. Observe for the combination of sepsis, inordinate pain, and unilateral edema. Crepitance is not a reliable indicator, and its absence does not rule out this diagnosis. The source is frequently polymicrobial, involving Clostridium and group A β-hemolytic Streptococcus. Gas in the subcutaneous tissue on computed tomography, and magnetic resonance imaging can help an evaluation, if the diagnosis is unclear. As stated earlier, the mainstays of treatment are aggressive debridement along with broad-spectrum antibiotics. Extensive debridement may require the assistance of gynecology oncology or surgery.

Wound Preparations and Dressings

There are several wound dressing types to choose from (**Table 3**) and topical agents to promote healing (**Box 6**). A popular technique is frequent wet to dry dressing changes, because they actively debride the unhealthy tissue. As a drawback, they are associated with increased patient discomfort, debride healthy tissue as well, and an incision should not be allowed to dry. Other dressing options include hydrogels and gauzes impregnated with antiseptics like iodine, chlorhexadine, and honey, which can maintain wound moisture without debriding healing tissue. Alginates have both antibacterial and hemostatic activity. Enzymatic agents like collagenase may be added to areas of nonviable tissue to break them down.[28] Care should be taken to avoid cytotoxic agents like full-strength betadine and hydrogen peroxide, because these indiscriminately destroy pathogens as well as healthy tissue, delaying healing.[29] A Cochrane review[70] did not show that one dressing or topical agent improved healing speed more than another.

Negative pressure wound therapy is being used increasingly. It acts as an occlusive dressing. By applying a sponge material with 400-μm to 600-μm micropores to the wound, with the application of intermittent or continuous suction, this system should remove excess effluent and promote the ingrowth of healthy tissue. Benefits include

Table 3
Dressing choices

Product	Advantages	Disadvantages	Indications	Comment
Gauzes	Inexpensive, accessible	Drying, poor barrier	Packing deep wounds	Change every 12–24 h
Films	Moisture retentive, transparent, semiocclusive protects wound from contamination	No absorption, fluid trapping, skin stripping	Wounds with minimal exudate, secondary dressing	Can leave in place $\leq$7 d or until fluid leaks
Hydrogels	Moisture retentive, nontraumatic removal, pain relief	May overhydrate	Dry wounds, painful wounds	Change every 1–3 d
Hydrocolloids	Long wear time, absorbent, occlusive, protects wound from contamination	Opaque, fluid trapping, skin stripping, malodorous discharge	Wounds with light moderate exudate	Can leave in place $\leq$7 d or until fluid leaks
Alginates and hydrofibers	Highly absorbent, hemostatic	Fibrous debris, lateral wicking (alginates only)	Wounds with moderate to heavy exudate mild hemostasis	Can leave in place until soaked with exudate
Foams	Absorbent, thermal insulation, occlusive	Opaque, malodorous discharge	Wounds with light to moderate exudate	Change every 3 d

From Wild T, Rahbarnia A, Kellner M. et al. Basics in nutrition and wound healing. Nutrition 2010;26(9):862–6; with permission.

Box 6
Topical agents

Topical antibiotics (eg, neomycin, bacitracin, mupirocin, polymyxin B, gentamycin)

Topical antiseptics (eg, povidone-iodine and chlorhexidine)

Topical steroid preparations (including antibiotic combinations)

Topical estrogen

Topical enzymatic agents

Topical growth factors

Topical collagen

Adapted from Vermeulen H, Ubbink D, Goossens A, et al. Dressings and topical agents for surgical wounds healing by secondary intention. Cochrane Database Syst Rev 2004;(2):3. CD003554.

---

decreased edema, decreased bacterial contamination, and promotion of wound contraction. There are minimal obstetric data regarding the outcomes of such wound management. One case series[71] showed promise in gynecology oncology patients with complex wound failures.

Reclosure

Wechter and colleagues[72] reviewed 8 prospective studies evaluating reclosure of disrupted laparotomy incisions. Closure with an en bloc technique was used in 6 of the studies, beginning 3 cm from the wound edge, incorporating the full wound thickness and exiting from the other edge. Suture materials used included polypropylene and nylon, which were removed on postoperative day 10. Overall success rate in reclosure was 81% to 100%. For patients with recurrent abscesses, they were reopened and allowed to heal by secondary intention. Secondary reclosure resulted in faster healing times (16–23 days vs 61–72).

Nutrition

Nutritional evaluation is a component of the workup for patients with chronic wounds and pressure ulcers, especially those at the greatest risk (eg, elderly, low socioeconomic status, and patients with malignancy). Up to 50% of medical and surgical patients in an urban setting may be malnourished.[38] Although the admitted obstetric patients are younger and healthier than the hospitalized medicine and surgical patients, they remain susceptible to malnutrition. This situation may occur because of increased metabolic needs from lactation, in combination with a postpartum complication like puerperal infection or from extended hospitalization.

Malnutrition should be considered in a wound with impaired healing, because it trumps the healing abilities of bedside dressings and wound care.[28] Inadequate nutrition may predate the wound or result from a complex wound. Wounds create a catabolic state because of increased energy demand. Carbohydrates are the primary source of energy, and larger, complicated wounds can have a significant impact on daily caloric requirements. Providing adequate glucose prevents muscle catabolism for gluconeogenesis.[38] For healthy adults, the recommended daily intake for protein is 0.8 g/kg/d, but this increases up to 2 g/kg/d for severely catabolic patients.[30]

The amino acids arginine and glutamine have been advocated for supplementation in wound healing. Arginine is a factor in collagen synthesis, growth factor release, and

> **Box 7**
> **Nutrition recommendations**
>
> Provide diet with appropriate caloric increase and additional protein
>
> Suspect malnourishment (acute or chronic) if delayed healing or friable, pale wound bed
>
> Evaluate serum markers for nutritional status
>
> Leading indicators (check weekly)
>
> Serum transferrin, prealbumin
>
> Lagging indicator (check monthly)
>
> Serum albumin
>
> Have a low threshold to consult nutrition for assistance optimizing diet and supplements (eg, micronutrients and vitamins)
>
> Consider alternative forms of nutritional intake if patient is unable to maintain caloric intake independently (eg, enteral feeding tube or total parental nutrition)

T-cell stimulation. Glutamine is involved in nucleotide formation and gluconeogenesis. Administration of these amino acids for wound care has shown mixed results.[30,38]

Several other vitamin and micronutrients including vitamin C, vitamin E, and zinc have been implicated in improved wound outcomes, but data on their efficacy are limited.[30,38]

Overall, obstetricians should be cognizant of the potential setbacks from nutritional deficiencies. Recommendations when assessing a poorly healing wound are listed in **Box 7**.

SUMMARY

SSIs after cesarean delivery are an economic burden and threat to the health of the obstetric population. There is a wide array of modifiable risks, ranging from patient-derived comorbidities to intrapartum factors. Recognizing these risks and targeting therapy accordingly can reduce postcesarean complications. Antibiotic prophylaxis is a vital universal intervention for cesarean delivery. For those who develop an SSI, therapy involves patient supportive care and optimizing the healing environment, along with wound care using various debridement techniques and topical agents supplemented by systemic antibiotics in selected cases.

Considering that the preponderance of evidence is limited at best, there are a multitude of opportunities for research in the future to address questions relating to optimal prevention and treatment strategies.

REFERENCES

1. Horan TC, Gaynes RP, Martone WJ, et al. CDC definitions of nosocomial surgical site infections, 1992: a modification of CDC definitions of surgical wound infections. Infect Control Hosp Epidemiol 1992;13:606–8.
2. Magill SS, Edwards JR, Bamberg W, et al. Emerging infections program healthcare-associated infections and antimicrobial use prevalence survey team. Multistate point-prevalence survey of health care-associated infections. N Engl J Med 2014;370:1198–208.
3. Cataife G, Weinberg DA, Wong HH, et al. The effect of Surgical Care Improvement Project (SCIP) compliance on surgical site infections (SSI). Med Care 2014;52:S66–73.

4. Martin JA, Hamilton BE, Ventura SJ, et al. Births: final data for 2012. Natl Vital Stat Rep 2013;62:1–87.
5. Opøien HK, Valbø A, Grinde-Andersen A, et al. Post-cesarean surgical site infections according to CDC standards: rates and risk factors. A prospective cohort study. Acta Obstet Gynecol Scand 2007;86:1097–102.
6. Olsen MA, Butler AM, Willers DM, et al. Risk factors for surgical site infection after low transverse cesarean section. Infect Control Hosp Epidemiol 2008;29: 477–84.
7. Chaim W, Bashiri A, Bar-David J, et al. Prevalence and clinical significance of postpartum endometritis and wound infection. Infect Dis Obstet Gynecol 2000;8:77–82.
8. Charrier L, Serafini P, Ribatti A, et al. Post-partum surgical wound infections: incidence after caesarean section in an Italian hospital. J Prev Med Hyg 2009;50:159–63.
9. Schneid-Kofman N, Sheiner E, Levy A, et al. Risk factors for wound infection following cesarean deliveries. Int J Gynaecol Obstet 2005;90:10–5.
10. Tran TS, Jamulitrat S, Chongsuvivatwong V, et al. Risk factors for postcesarean surgical site infection. Obstet Gynecol 2000;95:367–71.
11. Wloch C, Wilson J, Lamagni T, et al. Risk factors for surgical site infection following caesarean section in England: results from a multicentre cohort study. BJOG 2012;119:1324–33.
12. Gibbs RS. Clinical risk factors for puerperal infection. Obstet Gynecol 1980;55: 178S–84S.
13. Sachs BP, Yeh J, Acker D, et al. Cesarean section-related maternal mortality in Massachusetts, 1954-1985. Obstet Gynecol 1988;71:385–8.
14. Bodelon C, Bernabe-Ortiz A, Schiff MA, et al. Factors associated with peripartum hysterectomy. Obstet Gynecol 2009;114:115–23.
15. de Lissovoy G, Fraeman K, Hutchins V, et al. Surgical site infection: incidence and impact on hospital utilization and treatment costs. Am J Infect Control 2009;37:387–97.
16. Olsen MA, Butler AM, Willers DM, et al. Comparison of costs of surgical site infection and endometritis after cesarean delivery using claims and medical record data. Infect Control Hosp Epidemiol 2010;31:872–5.
17. Vermillion ST, Lamoutte C, Soper DE, et al. Wound infection after cesarean: effect of subcutaneous tissue thickness. Obstet Gynecol 2000;95:923–6.
18. Myles TD, Gooch J, Santolaya J. Obesity as an independent risk factor for infectious morbidity in patients who undergo cesarean delivery. Obstet Gynecol 2002;100:959–64.
19. Alanis MC, Villers MS, Law TL, et al. Complications of cesarean delivery in the massively obese parturient. Am J Obstet Gynecol 2010;203:271.e1–7.
20. Avila C, Bhangoo R, Figueroa R, et al. Association of smoking with wound complications after cesarean delivery. J Matern Fetal Neonatal Med 2012;25: 1250–3.
21. De Vivo A, Mancuso A, Giacobbe A, et al. Wound length and corticosteroid administration as risk factors for surgical-site complications following cesarean section. Acta Obstet Gynecol Scand 2010;89:355–9.
22. Emmons SL, Krohn M, Jackson M, et al. Development of wound infections among women undergoing cesarean section. Obstet Gynecol 1988;72: 559–64.
23. Henderson E, Love EJ. Incidence of hospital-acquired infections associated with caesarean section. J Hosp Infect 1995;29:245–55.

24. Killian CA, Graffunder EM, Vinciguerra TJ, et al. Risk factors for surgical-site infections following cesarean section. Infect Control Hosp Epidemiol 2001;22:613–7.
25. McLean M, Hines R, Polinkovsky M, et al. Type of skin incision and wound complications in the obese parturient. Am J Perinatol 2012;29:301–6.
26. Pelle H, Jepsen OB, Larsen SO, et al. Wound infection after cesarean section. Infect Control 1986;7:456–61.
27. Takoudes TC, Weitzen S, Slocum J, et al. Risk of cesarean wound complications in diabetic gestations. Am J Obstet Gynecol 2004;191:958–63.
28. Janis JE, Kwon RK, Lalonde DH. A practical guide to wound healing. Plast Reconstr Surg 2010;125:230e–44e.
29. Stadelmann WK, Digenis AG, Tobin GR. Impediments to wound healing. Am J Surg 1998;176:39S–47S.
30. Stechmiller JK. Understanding the role of nutrition and wound healing. Nutr Clin Pract 2010;25:61–8.
31. Alexander JM, Leveno KJ, Rouse DJ, et al. National Institute of Child Health and Human Development (NICHD) Maternal-Fetal Medicine Units Network (MFMU). Comparison of maternal and infant outcomes from primary cesarean delivery during the second compared with first stage of labor. Obstet Gynecol 2007;109:917–21.
32. Spong CY, Berghella V, Wenstrom KD, et al. Preventing the first cesarean delivery: summary of a joint Eunice Kennedy Shriver National Institute of Child Health and Human Development, Society for Maternal-Fetal Medicine, and American College of Obstetricians and Gynecologists Workshop. Obstet Gynecol 2012;120:1181–93.
33. Cetin A, Cetin M. Superficial wound disruption after cesarean delivery: effect of the depth and closure of subcutaneous tissue. Int J Gynaecol Obstet 1997;57:17–21.
34. Chelmow D, Rodriguez EJ, Sabatini MM. Suture closure of subcutaneous fat and wound disruption after cesarean delivery: a meta-analysis. Obstet Gynecol 2004;103:974–80.
35. Tipton AM, Cohen SA, Chelmow D. Wound infection in the obese pregnant woman. Semin Perinatol 2011;35:345–9.
36. Gates S, Anderson ER. Wound drainage for caesarean section. Cochrane Database Syst Rev 2013;(12):CD004549.
37. Hellums EK, Lin MG, Ramsey PS. Prophylactic subcutaneous drainage for prevention of wound complications after cesarean delivery–a metaanalysis. Am J Obstet Gynecol 2007;197:229–35.
38. Arnold M, Barbul A. Nutrition and wound healing. Plast Reconstr Surg 2006;117:42S–58S.
39. Wicke C, Halliday B, Allen D, et al. Effects of steroids and retinoids on wound healing. Arch Surg 2000;135:1265–70.
40. Munn MB, Rouse DJ, Owen J. Intraoperative hypothermia and post-cesarean wound infection. Obstet Gynecol 1998;91(4):582–4.
41. American College of Obstetricians and Gynecologists. ACOG practice bulletin No. 120: use of prophylactic antibiotics in labor and delivery. Obstet Gynecol 2011;117:1472–83.
42. Tita AT, Rouse DJ, Blackwell S, et al. Emerging concepts in antibiotic prophylaxis for cesarean delivery: a systematic review. Obstet Gynecol 2009;113:675–82.
43. Smaill FM, Gyte GM. Antibiotic prophylaxis versus no prophylaxis for preventing infection after cesarean section. Cochrane Database Syst Rev 2010;(1):CD007482.

44. Alfirevic Z, Gyte GM, Dou L. Different classes of antibiotics given to women routinely for preventing infection at caesarean section. Cochrane Database Syst Rev 2010;(10):CD008726.

45. Pevzner L, Swank M, Krepel C, et al. Effects of maternal obesity on tissue concentrations of prophylactic cefazolin during cesarean delivery. Obstet Gynecol 2011;117:877–82.

46. Dahlke JD, Mendez-Figueroa H, Rouse DJ, et al. Evidence-based surgery for cesarean delivery: an updated systematic review. Am J Obstet Gynecol 2013; 209:294–306.

47. Hadiati DR, Hakimi M, Nurdiati DS. Skin preparation for preventing infection following caesarean section. Cochrane Database Syst Rev 2012;(9):CD007462.

48. Darouiche RO, Wall MJ Jr, Itani KM, et al. Chlorhexidine-alcohol versus povidone-iodine for surgical-site antisepsis. N Engl J Med 2010;362:18–26.

49. Haas DM, Morgan S, Contreras K. Vaginal preparation with antiseptic solution before cesarean section for preventing postoperative infections. Cochrane Database Syst Rev 2013;(1):CD007892.

50. Duff P. A simple checklist for preventing major complications associated with cesarean delivery. Obstet Gynecol 2010;116:1393–6.

51. Ramsey PS, White AM, Guinn DA, et al. Subcutaneous tissue reapproximation, alone or in combination with drain, in obese women undergoing cesarean delivery. Obstet Gynecol 2005;105:967–73.

52. Walter CJ, Dumville JC, Sharp CA, et al. Systematic review and meta-analysis of wound dressings in the prevention of surgical-site infections in surgical wounds healing by primary intention. Br J Surg 2012;99:1185–94.

53. Connery SA, Downes KL, Young C. A retrospective study evaluating silver-impregnated dressings on cesarean wound healing. Adv Skin Wound Care 2012;25:414–9.

54. Hudson DA, Adams KG, Huyssteen AV, et al. Simplified negative pressure wound therapy: clinical evaluation of an ultraportable, no-canister system. Int Wound J 2013. [Epub ahead of print].

55. Webster J, Scuffham P, Sherriff KL, et al. Negative pressure wound therapy for skin grafts and surgical wounds healing by primary intention. Cochrane Database Syst Rev 2012;(4):CD009261.

56. Gibbs C, Orth T, Gerkovich M, et al. Traditional dressing compared with an external negative pressure system in preventing wound complications. Obstet Gynecol 2014;123(Suppl 1):145S.

57. Toon CD, Ramamoorthy R, Davidson BR, et al. Early versus delayed dressing removal after primary closure of clean and clean-contaminated surgical wounds. Cochrane Database Syst Rev 2013;(9):CD010259.

58. Toon CD, Sinha S, Davidson BR, et al. Early versus delayed post-operative bathing or showering to prevent wound complications. Cochrane Database Syst Rev 2013;(10):CD010075.

59. Wild T, Rahbarnia A, Kellner M, et al. Basics in nutrition and wound healing. Nutrition 2010;26:862–6.

60. Li J, Chen J, Kirsner R. Pathophysiology of acute wound healing. Clin Dermatol 2007;25:9–18.

61. Roberts S, Maccato M, Faro S, et al. The microbiology of post-cesarean wound morbidity. Obstet Gynecol 1993;81:383–6.

62. Andrews WW, Shah SR, Goldenberg RL, et al. Association of post-cesarean delivery endometritis with colonization of the chorioamnion by *Ureaplasma urealyticum*. Obstet Gynecol 1995;85:509–14.

63. Owen J, Andrews WW. Wound complications after cesarean sections. Clin Obstet Gynecol 1994;37:842–55.
64. Cunningham FG, Leveno KJ, Bloom SL, et al, editors. Williams obstetrics. 24th edition. New York: McGraw-Hill; 2014.
65. Mudge EJ. Recent accomplishments in wound healing. Int Wound J 2014. [Epub ahead of print].
66. Smith F, Dryburgh N, Donaldson J, et al. Debridement for surgical wounds. Cochrane Database Syst Rev 2013;(9):CD006214.
67. McNeeley SG Jr, Hendrix SL, Bennett SM, et al. Synthetic graft placement in the treatment of fascial dehiscence with necrosis and infection. Am J Obstet Gynecol 1998;179:1430–4.
68. Goepfert AR, Guinn DA, Andrews WW, et al. Necrotizing fasciitis after cesarean delivery. Obstet Gynecol 1997;89:409–12.
69. Gallup DG, Meguiar RV. Coping with necrotizing fasciitis. Contemp Ob Gyn 2004;49:38.
70. Vermeulen H, Ubbink D, Goossens A, et al. Dressings and topical agents for surgical wounds healing by secondary intention. Cochrane Database Syst Rev 2004;(2):CD003554.
71. Argenta PA, Rahaman J, Gretz HF 3rd, et al. Vacuum-assisted closure in the treatment of complex gynecologic wound failures. Obstet Gynecol 2002;99:497–501.
72. Wechter ME, Pearlman MD, Hartmann KE. Reclosure of the disrupted laparotomy wound: a systematic review. Obstet Gynecol 2005;106:376–83.

Index

Note: Page numbers of article titles are in **boldface** type.

A

AIDS
  described, 548
Antibiotics
  in chorioamnionitis management, 660
  in postcesarean SSI management, 681–682

B

Breastfeeding
  HIV in pregnancy and, 561

C

Cesarean wound infection, **671–689**. *See also* Surgical site infection (SSI),
  postcesarean
Chorioamnionitis, **649–669**
  clinical outcomes of, 654–657
  complications of, 661–664
  concerns about, 661–664
  described, 650–651
  discussion, 664–665
  future directions in, 664–665
  GBS and, 653–654
  introduction, 649–650
  management of, 657–661
    antibiotics in, 660
    neonatal, 660–661
  Mycoplasma and *Ureaplasma* spp. and, 618–619
  prevalence/incidence/mortality rates, 653
  risk factors for, 651–653
CMV. *See* Cytomegalovirus (CMV)
Congenital CMV, **593–599**. *See also* Cytomegalovirus (CMV), congenital
Contraception
  HIV–related, 562
Corticosteroid(s)
  postcesarean SSI related to, 675
Counseling
  preconception
    HIV–related, 552–554
Cytomegalovirus (CMV)
  biology of, 594
  congenital, **593–599**

Obstet Gynecol Clin N Am 41 (2014) 691–697
http://dx.doi.org/10.1016/S0889-8545(14)00091-6
0889-8545/14/$ – see front matter © 2014 Elsevier Inc. All rights reserved.

obgyn.theclinics.com

United States Postal Service

Statement of Ownership, Management, and Circulation
(All Periodicals Publications Except Requestor Publications)

1. Publication Title	2. Publication Number	3. Filing Date
Obstetrics and Gynecology Clinics of North America	0 0 0 - 2 7 6	9/14/14

4. Issue Frequency	5. Number of Issues Published Annually	6. Annual Subscription Price
Mar, Jun, Sep, Dec	4	$310.00

7. Complete Mailing Address of Known Office of Publication (Not printer) (Street, city, county, state, and ZIP+4®)

Elsevier Inc.
360 Park Avenue South
New York, NY 10010-1710

Contact Person: Stephen R. Bushing

Telephone (Include area code): 215-239-3688

8. Complete Mailing Address of Headquarters or General Business Office of Publisher (Not printer)

Elsevier Inc., 360 Park Avenue South, New York, NY 10010-1710

9. Full Names and Complete Mailing Addresses of Publisher, Editor, and Managing Editor (Do not leave blank)

Publisher (Name and complete mailing address)

Linda Belfus, Elsevier Inc., 1600 John F. Kennedy Blvd., Suite 1800, Philadelphia, PA 19103-2899

Editor (Name and complete mailing address)

Kerry Holland, Elsevier Inc., 1600 John F. Kennedy Blvd., Suite 1800, Philadelphia, PA 19103-2899

Managing Editor (Name and complete mailing address)

Adrianne Brigido, Elsevier Inc., 1600 John F. Kennedy Blvd., Suite 1800, Philadelphia, PA 19103-2899

10. Owner (Do not leave blank. If the publication is owned by a corporation, give the name and address of the corporation immediately followed by the names and addresses of all stockholders owning or holding 1 percent or more of the total amount of stock. If not owned by a corporation, give the names and addresses of the individual owners. If owned by a partnership or other unincorporated firm, give its name and address as well as those of each individual owner. If the publication is published by a nonprofit organization, give its name and address.)

Full Name	Complete Mailing Address
Wholly owned subsidiary of	1600 John F. Kennedy Blvd, Ste. 1800
Reed/Elsevier, US holdings	Philadelphia, PA 19103-2899

11. Known Bondholders, Mortgagees, and Other Security Holders Owning or Holding 1 Percent or More of Total Amount of Bonds, Mortgages, or Other Securities. If none, check box. ☐ None

Full Name	Complete Mailing Address
N/A	

12. Tax Status (For completion by nonprofit organizations authorized to mail at nonprofit rates) (Check one)

The purpose, function, and nonprofit status of this organization and the exempt status for federal income tax purposes:
☐ Has Not Changed During Preceding 12 Months
☐ Has Changed During Preceding 12 Months (Publisher must submit explanation of change with this statement)

PS Form 3526, August 2012 (Page 1 of 3 (Instructions Page 3)) PSN 7530-01-000-9931 PRIVACY NOTICE: See our Privacy policy in www.usps.com

13. Publication Title	14. Issue Date for Circulation Data Below
Obstetrics and Gynecology Clinics of North America	September 2014

15. Extent and Nature of Circulation			Average No. Copies Each Issue During Preceding 12 Months	No. Copies of Single Issue Published Nearest to Filing Date
a. Total Number of Copies (Net press run)			880	917
b. Paid Circulation (By Mail and Outside the Mail)	(1)	Mailed Outside-County Paid Subscriptions Stated on PS Form 3541. (Include paid distribution above nominal rate, advertiser's proof copies, and exchange copies)	345	406
	(2)	Mailed In-County Paid Subscriptions Stated on PS Form 3541 (Include paid distribution above nominal rate, advertiser's proof copies, and exchange copies)		
	(3)	Paid Distribution Outside the Mails Including Sales Through Dealers and Carriers, Street Vendors, Counter Sales, and Other Paid Distribution Outside USPS®	243	257
	(4)	Paid Distribution by Other Classes Mailed Through the USPS (e.g. First-Class Mail®)		
c. Total Paid Distribution (Sum of 15b (1), (2), (3), and (4))			588	663
d. Free or Nominal Rate Distribution (By Mail and Outside the Mail)	(1)	Free or Nominal Rate Outside-County Copies Included on PS Form 3541	46	54
	(2)	Free or Nominal Rate In-County Copies Included on PS Form 3541		
	(3)	Free or Nominal Rate Copies Mailed at Other Classes Through the USPS (e.g. First-Class Mail)		
	(4)	Free or Nominal Rate Distribution Outside the Mail (Carriers or other means)		
e. Total Free or Nominal Rate Distribution (Sum of 15d (1), (2), (3) and (4))			46	54
f. Total Distribution (Sum of 15c and 15e)			634	717
g. Copies not Distributed (See instructions to publishers #4 (page #3))			246	200
h. Total (Sum of 15f and g)			880	917
i. Percent Paid (15c divided by 15f times 100)			92.74%	92.47%

16. Total circulation includes electronic copies. Report circulation on PS Form 3526-X worksheet.

17. Publication of Statement of Ownership
If the publication is a general publication, publication of this statement is required. Will be printed in the December 2014 issue of this publication.

18. Signature and Title of Editor, Publisher, Business Manager, or Owner

Stephen R. Bushing – Inventory Distribution Coordinator

Date: September 14, 2014

I certify that all information furnished on this form is true and complete. I understand that anyone who furnishes false or misleading information on this form or who omits material or information requested on the form may be subject to criminal sanctions (including fines and imprisonment) and/or civil sanctions (including civil penalties).

PS Form 3526, August 2012 (Page 2 of 3)

Printed and bound by CPI Group (UK) Ltd, Croydon, CR0 4YY

03/10/2024

01040487-0017